WELLNESS
in MIND

Your Brain's Surprising Secrets to Gaining Health from the Inside Out

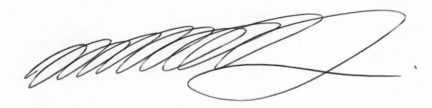

By

M. ANDREW GARRISON, M.S. CPT HC

with

SALLY K. SEVERINO, M.D.

ISBN: 978-1-4834-4264-8 (sc)
ISBN: 978-1-4834-4263-1 (hc)
ISBN: 978-1-4834-4265-5 (e)

Library of Congress Control Number: 2015919697

Lulu Publishing Services rev. date: 12/17/2015

To my mother
Cecilia Castillo Garrison (1943-1987)
To my big brother
Daniel Ray Garrison III (1968-2013)

—— M. Andrew Garrison

To my two grand daughters-in-law
Cadence Connelly Peery
Irelynn Connelly Peery

—— Sally K. Severino

ENDORSEMENTS

Advance praise for Wellness In Mind

"A powerful message is being given here—how to move beyond our roles, personas, and what we do in life, to living authentically from a place called beingness. The potential for healing disappointments, setbacks, and even traumas is available to us from this place of Being in relationship or "resonance" with others. Andrew's personal story of physical and emotional healing after an amputation inspires and motivates us to learn about how living from our Being Image heals our sense of separation and brings fulfillment to every area of life. It's time, the authors suggest, that we leave behind our normal preoccupation with Self Image (comparing ourselves to others) and Body Image (competing with others) and know that true Self-Esteem comes from engaging in a 'collaborative co-creating' of each other and our communities in wellness and health. It is by living from our Being Image, then, that we achieve true fulfillment, inner peace and enduring love."

> Gail Carr Feldman, PhD, LLC, author of *Midlife Crash Course: The Journey from Crisis to Full Creative Power*

"As an assistant coach for seventeen years in the National Football League and Head Coach for eight years at two NCAA Division 1 Football programs, I immediately recognized philosophical parallels between my coaching experiences and the layered approach of Wellness In Mind. The authors champion knowledge as the basis of informed change with regard to exercise programs and dieting. They continue by stimulating healing life strategies through self-reflection and ultimately complete the wellness journey by accessing our desire for healthy relationships. I recommend Wellness In Mind for anyone seeking to tap into their innate ability to create healthy surroundings with and through others—to rewrite destiny as the sole owner of their wellness."

> Mike Sheppard, 37-year College/NFL Coach

"M. Andrew Garrison and Sally K. Severino, M.D apply the latest knowledge in neuroscience to a valuable discussion of how we function in the most important areas of our lives. Dr. Severino's work on the mother-infant dyad leads to the emphasis on utilizing our inborn needs and wiring to connect with one another, to live fuller, enriched lives. Andrew Garrison builds on this foundation a new approach and extremely useful guide to understanding how we can reach higher levels of functioning in physical, occupational, social, intellectual and spiritual aspects of our lives. Utilizing the principles in this book will improve your life!"

Barry M. Panter, MD, PhD.
Clinical Professor of Psychiatry (emeritus) University of
Southern California School of Medicine
Co-Editor and Co-Author, *Creativity and Madness: Psychological Studies of Art and Artists*. Volumes 1 and 2.

Contents

Foreword xi
Introduction xiii

PART I – INFORMATION: WELLNESS KNOWLEDGE TO TRANSFORM YOUR HEALTH

Chapter 1: What is Being Image, Anyway? 3
Chapter 2: Move It! 18
Chapter 3: No More Starving! Fuel Yourself with Food and Love 26

PART II – INTROSPECTION: KNOW YOURSELF TO ENHANCE YOUR WELLNESS HABITS

Chapter 4: Wellness: It's All in Your Head 39
Chapter 5: Bullseye! Target Well-Being for Life 48
Chapter 6: REACH for Resilience! 56

PART III – INTERSUBJECTIVITY: PLAY WELL WITH OTHERS TO CO-CREATE LIFE AND HEALTH

Chapter 7: Serving Wellness to Others 69
Chapter 8: Wellness in the World 79

APPENDIX: More of the Science Behind Wellness in Mind 91
Wellness in Mind Activities 103
Acknowledgements 113
Notes 115
References 119

Foreword

With the title, *Wellness in Mind: Your Brain's Surprising Secrets to Gaining Health from the Inside Out*, the reader presumably expects to learn about the mind-body connection and its important role in promoting wellness. This book delivers on those expectations. Written by M. Andrew Garrison and Sally K. Severino, MD, a well-respected exercise professional and a noted psychiatrist, respectively, *Wellness in Mind* challenges paradigms related to current concepts of wellness. They offer a new, hopeful approach for those seeking that ever-elusive state of true wellness. The authors focus on a concept they call "Being Image," which suggests that our focus should shift from self to others, from competition to collaboration and, ultimately from doing (achieving) to being. With a style that is clear, concise, and engaging, the authors review the keys to healthier, well living in a way that is profoundly simple and straightforward. Each chapter of the book addresses a single aspect of health and wellness with the aim of helping readers bolster their Being Images. Finally, a number of truly inspiring stories and interactive exercises are shared throughout the book that bring many of the concepts to life to help translate them into practice. In short, *Wellness in Mind* is must reading for anyone interested in protecting their most valuable asset—their health.

Cedric X. Bryant, Ph.D., FACSM
Chief Science Officer
American Council on Exercise
San Diego, CA

Introduction

We are on the verge of a wellness revolution, poised to explode all the old myths and habits that keep us stuck in feeling not-good-enough, stressed, and unhealthy. We now know that we can harness the power of our brain to become healthier, happier, and more whole than we could ever have imagined—and this book is your guide.

Wellness in Mind: Your Brain's Surprising Secrets to Gaining Health from the Inside Out is a simple manual to help you uncover true wellness. We've included worksheets, exercises and quizzes, hints for giving your attitudes a makeover, inspiring personal stories—even two power-food recipes! And it's all based on the latest scientific research.

Here's the crux: our usual approach to health is based on a lie. This lie permeates our culture, and it manifests in today's world problems, such as the widening gap between those few who have and those many who have not, relationships that treat persons as things, and threats to the availability of healthy food, water, and air. *The lie is that human beings are isolated individuals.*

The latest social, psychological, and neuroscientific research points to the real truth that we are not just individuals: we are collaborative co-creators of one another. We can only come into our true humanity, not in individualistic competition or comparison with others, but in collaboration.

The current paradigms around wellness are based on old concepts of body image that feed the lie of isolation, with its endless quest for physiological success. The truth is, consumerism and the interests of big business keep the whole miserable machine running. Ads tell us we need the newest exercise gadget or the current fad diet to build a body that will get us the job we want or the love we seek. Think about it: if we already believed we were adequate as is, nobody would buy any widgets or diet books or products, and a multibillion-dollar industry would tank in a nanosecond. As far as advertisers are concerned, we will never be perfect, because then we wouldn't spend our money on their stuff. Only looking and performing better than others will feed our self-esteem, which sets up an unhappy cycle of rivalry and feeling less-than.

The Wellness in Mind approach is very different. It focuses on something we like to call Being Image. Being Image is not just the way we look or the way we compare with others, it is our whole person *in relation* to others. Being Image honors interconnectedness. When we hold our Being Image in mind rather than staying locked in body image, we move out of less-than thinking and into a liberating, humanizing sense of relationship and positivity. Being Image gives us hope. When we center our being—especially our being in relationships—we focus not on what we think we have to achieve but on who we truly are and who we can become.

Every person has a unique and valuable Being Image. When we experience each other's being, we discover and harness the body's inner urge to wellness and connect with our human birthright of greater vitality and health.

Wellness in Mind offers a three-part approach (information, introspection, and intersubjectivity) to transform the way you feel about yourself and your health—and will help you to achieve the most vibrant health possible. In Part I (information), you will learn the groundbreaking knowledge—based on the latest scientific research—to help you build vital new wellness skills. Part II (introspection) invites you to do a little self-examination, looking inside to recognize habits that may be undermining your health and offering techniques to form healthier new ones. And Part III (intersubjectivity) emphasizes the exciting ways we can co-create wellness with and through each other.

Every chapter of Wellness in Mind focuses on one aspect of health and wellness, helping you to strengthen your Being Image. We include lots of inspiring true stories that illustrate helpful ways in which others have put each chapter's recommendations into practice.

PART I – INFORMATION: WELLNESS KNOWLEDGE TO TRANSFORM YOUR HEALTH

Chapter 1 – First we explain the basic concepts of Being Image and wellness, starting with the attachment patterns formed in your infancy that still affect you today. We include an easy-to-remember acronym that will allow you to keep Wellness in Mind and a true story that left Andrew an amputee after a motorcycle accident. Andrew learned how his relationships with others and his own Being Image were instrumental in his achieving wellness.

To reframe the concept of wellness we have to understand the difference between need and desire, so we'll introduce you to scientific research that supports interconnection as a key to healing and wellness. Andrew shares more about his post-accident healing journey, including how he reframed the incident and embraced interconnection to discover his own wellness in the process. Then we'll give you an activity sheet so you can begin to define your own Being Image through life values, your vision, and your mission, which make up the underlying blueprint for all your wellness choices.

Chapter 2 – Our bodies love to move. When we stop viewing exercise as a chore, but start seeing it as a pleasure, we honor our whole being. We'll help you to recognize and accept your body type, understand the role of exercise in your life, evaluate physical fitness according to your Being Image, and then set attainable fitness goals that are actually satisfying. Learn the FITT Principle for success and discover the latest in contemporary fitness training!

Chapter 3 – Nurture your Being Image with foods that are enjoyable to eat. We'll boost your critical thinking skills and help you recognize the three major ingredients in processed and fast foods that undermine your health when eaten in excess. You'll be introduced to nutrient-dense foods that nurture your whole person. Eating is a delicious part of your Being Image!

PART II – INTROSPECTION: KNOW YOURSELF AND ENHANCE YOUR WELLNESS HABITS

Chapter 4 – Is your unconscious holding you back? Most of us have blind spots that can cause us to suffer. Here we will identify coping mechanisms that have become barriers to wellness and help you transform the burdens of the past by taking loving action in the present.

Chapter 5 – Become the Chief Executive Officer (CEO) of your life and learn the simple steps to target your well-being plan. We include helpful worksheets for setting SMART goals and doing a SWOT analysis, so you can hit the bullseye.

Chapter 6 – Respond to the triggers of eating unhealthy with the acronym REACH by keeping meaningful thoughts and actions within arm's reach. You'll also face the fears that hold you back from achieving the wellness you deserve—in seven simple steps.

PART III – INTERSUBJECTIVITY: PLAY WELL WITH OTHERS TO CO-CREATE LIFE AND HEALTH

Chapter 7 – Share your wellness with others for happier, healthier relationships. Here we'll help you to discover your own relational consciousness that embraces families, workplaces, and communities. The gift of wellness keeps on giving!

Chapter 8 – Find out the six settings where you can share your wellness with the world. Then read a few wise words to empower and encourage you as you fully embrace your well-being, becoming a worthy model for others to imitate.

We invite you to take the Wellness in Mind journey with us toward more vibrant health by honoring your Being Image and fostering happier, more respectful, and collaborative relationships. We hope you will take our science-based program to heart, benefit from it, and thrive! It all starts in your head.

PART I

INFORMATION: WELLNESS KNOWLEDGE TO TRANSFORM YOUR HEALTH

This section, based on the latest scientific research, will give you the vocabulary and factual data you need to keep Wellness in Mind.

Chapter 1

What is Being Image, Anyway?

> Bad things do happen; how I respond to them defines my character and the quality of my life. I can choose to sit in perpetual sadness, immobilized by the gravity of my loss, or I can choose to rise from the pain and treasure the most precious gift I have—life itself.
>
> —Walter Anderson

We are all familiar with body image. Body image is what we see as our physical self in comparison to others and can be characterized as judgment based on external appearance. The body image sold in American culture puts us in deficit-mode functioning as we strive to make our bodies conform to an ideal image. But since perfection is an impossible dream, we can never get there. In fact, a multibillion-dollar health and beauty industry is built on our stampede to buy anything that promises a better, stronger, sexier body image that we can never attain. Self esteem suffers as we chase comparisons that breed concern and worry about our talents, abilities and appearance. We limit our *beingness*—a lived body-mind-spirit knowing—as we distract our goodness by constantly feeling less-than somebody.

Being Image is different. It goes beyond what we see and think in comparison with others. Being Image is how we experience our body and self through interaction with others.

Body Image: What we see in comparison.

Being Image: How we experience in collaboration.

Being Image begins with our earliest caregivers. Here's how the process unfolds: an infant's face expresses his or her feelings. When a caregiver sees the baby's facial expressions, the caregiver's brain lights up as if they were feeling the same emotion as the infant. Now, the caregiver's face expresses the feeling and reflects it back to the baby. Seeing this emotional confirmation of their feelings, babies know in their very deepest being that they are seen and empathized with. In this process, our Being Image and our patterns of relating to others are born. In these early experiences of collaboration with others, we co-create each other by participating in each other's feelings.

Science has proven that humans do not exist in isolation; we are hardwired to connect with each other. We learn not by transferring knowledge, but by interacting with each other. This is how we co-create new being and new becoming. For more of the science behind this, see "Mirror Neurons: Why We Imitate Others" in the Appendix.

By the time we reach adulthood, the dynamics of our early formation have become our brain's default setting for our Being Image and for our relationship patterns. This default setting determines the way our nervous system physically and emotionally regulates our bodies within us and between us and others. It contributes to the view in our minds of *our* world, not *the* world and what is *actual, real and true*.

We may not know how the world works, but we *believe* that we know based on our personal knowledge and experiences, which are based on our attachment patterns that define our view of the world as either safe or dangerous. We carry our view of the world—our template for how to relate to others and our environment—with us into adulthood.

If we were fortunate enough to be reared by loving caregivers, our brains automatically know how to access wellness and activate health. But what if you were inadequately mirrored and nurtured? Unfortunately, that's the case with so many of us. Well, there is good news: no matter how abused, neglected, or misunderstood you have been, if you are alive to read this book, there is hope. Our brains can be retaught; we can learn how to access wellness and activate health in our Being Image and in our relationships.

Here's an inspiring true story about a real-life poor little rich girl that proves it.

A Story of Hope

Kelly is an attractive, willowy brunette from a wealthy family, educated in the finest schools, with a satisfying career as an art appraiser. But despite all of her seeming advantages, she had struggled for years with anxiety and severe depression. Gradually, her symptoms worsened and episodes of despair became almost paralyzing. After resisting therapy for years, she eventually gave in and began seeing Dr. Sally. Under Dr. Sally's guidance, Kelly began to remember her infancy and childhood. This turned out to be the key that would unlock her mystery.

"To everyone who knew me, it just didn't make sense why I would be so depressed," she says now. "I had everything—I'd gone to the best boarding schools, skiing in the Alps, shopping sprees in Paris, all that. I had a closet full of designer clothes, a beautiful home, work I loved. Yes, I'd had some really disappointing love affairs. Looking back, all the men had one trait in common—they seemed cold and distant. I had never found true love. But everything else in my life was great. What was the matter with me? Doctors had prescribed various drugs but nothing really seemed to help. I was at the end of my rope when I went to see Dr. Sally."

Together, they began to explore Kelly's past. The child of affluent career-obsessed parents, Kelly was born prematurely. "When I think about it now," Kelly says, "it almost felt like my mother's womb wasn't a safe place for me to be—as if she didn't want me there." In those days, the importance of nurturing touch for preemies wasn't the common knowledge it is now. Kelly was placed in an incubator and there she stayed, without any loving interaction from her parents at all, until she was ready to be discharged from the hospital.

"My theory is that the nurses must have given me some of the love I needed, or I don't think I'd be alive now," Kelly recalled. "My parents were so busy with their own lives, I wonder if they even remembered that they had a child. As soon as they brought me home from the hospital, they got a nanny for me." We don't know the nanny's backstory, only that she didn't believe in showing affection. "I guess she thought it would spoil me," Kelly remembered. "I don't think she ever hugged me. The only time she ever held me on her lap was when I got hurt and she had to put antibiotic cream on my cuts. Every once in awhile she'd say I was 'a good girl' if I did what I was told, but that was about it. She was big into discipline, but she didn't have any warmth or heart for me. Mine was a lonely childhood."

For many years, Kelly lived that classic poor little rich girl life, shunted from the nanny to one prestigious boarding school after another. "I loved school, at least—art history was my passion—and when I was finally grown up and on my own, I found work that I loved. I kept telling myself that I was fine, but I was having trouble sleeping—I had terrible nightmares—and sometimes I would go for days without eating. I lost so much weight that my menstrual periods ceased. Things were going from bad to worse.

"The big shift for me came in a session with Dr. Sally. She had asked me how I felt about my childhood and I was surprised how much pain I felt. In the past, I had denied my neglect; maybe I figured everybody was raised like that. Whatever the reason, I had no idea it would hurt so much.

"When I was finally done sharing my pain, it was really quiet in her office for awhile. I'll never forget what she said then because I could sense that it really came from her heart. She said, 'You deserved to be loved, Kelly. Someone should have held you and looked at you and sung lullabies to you and loved you.' That was when it really hit me—I had been missing this huge piece that every baby should have. I started crying and when I looked up, I saw that Dr. Sally had tears in her eyes, too. I think that was the beginning of healing for me—that someone really understood the root of all this pain I'd been feeling since before I could even talk."

This moment of what scientists refer to as "intersubjective resonance"—a technical term for deeply-felt empathy between people—was a turning point for Kelly. Over the course of several months, she was able to receive the positive re-parenting from Dr. Sally that she needed so badly. Together, they co-created new neural pathways in Kelly's brain and worked to reframe the old damaging memories of neglect into a healthy Being Image. Kelly went on to meet and marry a warm and deeply loving man, a far cry from the old paradigm of her unloving parents. Now she is thriving instead of simply surviving.

There is a miracle here, and it can be true for any of us. The miracle is twofold: first and foremost, it is never too late to receive the loving gaze that will heal and help us. And second, when we reframe and view the past differently, it creates actual structural and functional changes in our brains—changes that are just as real as if this more positive past were actually true. We can actually remake our pasts and ourselves.

When Kelly finally surrendered to her need for love, she recognized and owned her broken-heartedness. She became able to receive Dr. Sally's compassionate and loving attunement and form a loving Being Image. While it didn't happen overnight, and it did involve ongoing work with a trained therapist, the story of Kelly's healing is a beacon of hope for us all. It is never too late to be embraced in the great womb of compassion and be healed by our deep desire for love and nourishment. We can begin to have Wellness in Mind.

To learn more about this, see "Attachment Patterns: How Relationships Organize Our Nervous System" in the Appendix.

Dr. Bill Hettler of Texas A&M University and co-founder of the National Wellness Institute (NWI) presents wellness in a dynamic and holistic way. His approach to health takes into consideration all of our physical, mental, and social conditions. Seen in this way, wellness is a state of total well-being, a state of happiness, contentment, healthy beliefs about stress, overall good physical and mental health, and a good quality of life.[1] We agree with the overall definition of wellness that has long been used by NWI: *Wellness is an active process through which people become aware of, and make choices toward, a more successful existence.*

Dr. Hettler defines six dimensions of wellness, which form an interdependent model that provides the categories from which NWI derives its resources and services.[2] Remember the old nursery rhyme, "Ring around the rosie, a pocketful of posies"? Well, the six dimensions of wellness make the acronym **POSIES**, which will help you remember them. Here they are:

Physical wellness recognizes the need for regular physical activity. Physical development encourages learning about diet and nutrition while discouraging the use of tobacco, drugs, and excessive alcohol consumption.

Occupational wellness recognizes personal satisfaction and enrichment in our life through work. In other words, loving the work we do is a form of wellness.

Social wellness encourages contributing to our environment and community. It emphasizes the interdependence between people and nature and recognizes the fact that we are social animals: people are generally happier and healthier when they are in meaningful connection with others.

Intellectual wellness recognizes our creative, stimulating mental activities. Well people expand their knowledge and skills while discovering the potential for sharing their gifts with others.

Emotional wellness signifies the degree to which we feel positive and enthusiastic about our self and life. It involves the capacity to manage our feelings and related behaviors including the realistic assessment of our limitations, development of self-regulation, and ability to cope effectively with stress.

Spiritual wellness recognizes our search for meaning and purpose in human existence. It includes the development of a growing appreciation for the depth and expanse of life and natural forces that exist in the universe.

What does this mean for you? Wellness is a process of achieving full potential. You enter into it consciously, and it is self-directed and evolving. Wellness is multidimensional and holistic. It encompasses lifestyle, mental and spiritual well-being, and the environment. Wellness is positive and affirming.

POSIES isn't just a memorable acronym, it is a meaningful metaphor as well. A posy is a small collection of your favorite flowers. Each one is unique but together they contribute a rich bouquet of scents that remind you of life's beauty. All six dimensions of wellness overlap and profoundly affect each other, so positive change in one wellness dimension results in improvements in overall wellness, improvements in our relationships, and improvements in our very being.

For example, when we look at the physical wellness dimension, we already know it's better to consume foods and beverages that enhance good health and it's better to be physically fit than out of shape. But our state of mind about diet and exercise is also supremely important. Without tranquility, we tend to view exercise as work and diet as suffering. With inner peace, we are better able to honor our bodies by enjoying food and welcoming exercise.

The occupational wellness dimension may provide the most profound and diverse influence of all. Did you know that for most people work consumes half of their waking hours? Remembering this, we realize how important it is to use wellness strategies on the job. It's ideal when our work is consistent with our personal values, interests, and beliefs. But contributing our unique gifts, skills, and talents to our work place can bring about even greater personal satisfaction.

The social circles in which we move exert a huge influence on us within our social wellness dimension. That influence may be good, bad, or indifferent, so it's useful to take a nonjudgmental look to see if we need to optimize that influence, minimize it, or leave it alone. Ideally, the well person contributes to the common welfare of his or her community and lives in harmony with others and the environment.

The intellectual wellness dimension brings our mind into play. Using our brain, our mind also determines what we choose to learn, practice, master, or ignore. Holding a positive attitude of open curiosity is key to learning about others and utilizing our talents and skills to better the world.

The emotional wellness dimension registers how positive we feel about our thoughts. The well person accepts a wide range of feelings in themself and in others, expresses those feelings freely, and manages those feelings effectively. Rather than denying them, all feelings are honored. In fact, feelings are used to inform the mind so decision-making can move the person toward his or her Being Image. In other words, mind and emotions work in tandem.

Finally, the spiritual wellness dimension grounds us in beliefs that guide our daily actions. A well person lives with a sense of meaningfulness, in ways consistent with their values and beliefs. The well person lives with integrity and tolerance for the values and beliefs of others, resulting in relationships that exude wellness.

The development of our wellness is a lifelong process that involves personal time and commitment. It's also a moment-to-moment experience of our relationships with others and within ourselves. But how do we come to be who we are? What determines our beingness?

These questions bring us back to our Being Image. Our Being Image is the internalization of interrelated talents and passions. It is our mind's integration of many internal and external experiences. Its purpose is connecting with and serving each other and our community. And it is grounded in our human physiology and biology.

How exactly do we become aware of and embrace our Being Image? Here's how Andrew did it.

My Journey to Being Image

My wake-up call happened just four months after I had married the love of my life, Chamar. On September 25, 2008, I drove my Buell XB12R motorcycle to play in a recreation league flag football game. I didn't take time to put on motorcycle gear. I was dressed in T-shirt and shorts and wearing Nike sport sandals, the type athletes relax in when they get out of restrictive high-top cleats. I wasn't wearing a helmet.

The game was canceled. Disappointed, I dropped in to a Chili's restaurant, where I met up with a friend. We ate some fish and rice, watched a football game on TV, then left for home early in the fourth quarter. Heading west, I exited the freeway and encountered unusually thick traffic. I began strategizing how to swiftly maneuver through the congestion.

That's the last thing I remember.

When I woke up, I was in the Intensive Care Unit at the University of New Mexico Hospital. Chamar was there, adamant about staying with me overnight. She talked the hospital staff into allowing her a bed next to mine, confirming her commitment to me despite what had suddenly become an uncertain future.

I was in bad shape. The accident injured almost every body part that I had left unprotected. My head was lacerated front to back. I had six broken ribs and bruised lungs. My right clavicle was fractured and my left shoulder was torn. My left foot was heavily wrapped; the doctors tried their best to save it.

Six days later I left the hospital an amputee.

My journey to becoming aware of and embracing my Being Image began with love and continued with love. From Chamar's dedicated presence to a large number of phone calls, flowers, e-mails and visitors, I felt unconditionally loved. One visitor in particular pointed me in the direction of embracing my Being Image.

When he ambled into my hospital room, my cousin Ricky Garcia looked drawn and wan, and his clothes seemed too big for his body. Although he was only fifty-five years old, he looked much older. I will never forget his words to me that day, "Andrew, just take life slow. Don't do what I have done. I've always rushed through life and now I'm not feeling well. You need to place things in their proper perspective!"

The next weekend he was admitted to the hospital with stage IV stomach cancer and died three months later. When I rolled into the funeral in a wheelchair, my cousin Carla was straightforward, "After the scare you gave us, we would never have imagined that it would be Ricky we'd be burying."

My accident forced me to pause and reflect. Like most human beings, I had always identified myself primarily through my body image. In college, I was a Letterman in football at the University of New Mexico, a bodybuilding competitor, and a power lifter who once lifted 1,200 pounds in competition. Now, without my left foot, I experienced myself as handicapped. Thinking of myself as handicapped undermined my body image, which up to that point had only brought me temporary satisfaction through athletic competition.

I had to find a different way of viewing myself.

I had three choices. I could beat myself up, forever angry that I had behaved so carelessly on September 25th or I could cling to the mandates of our society where body image trumps Being Image as our primary road to wellness. Instead, I found a third way: I became aware that an emphasis on body image was an illusion; an emphasis on body image said "no" to the healing love I was experiencing from others. I realized that Being Image is primary; it results from saying "yes" to the outpouring of love.

Beingness requires no comparison to or competition against another. We all have a being—we just need to become aware of it in order to accept that we are loved. Then we can engage in a collaborative co-creating of each other, building each other up towards wellness and health.

Becoming aware of my Being Image opened me up. Because of it, I could embrace and enjoy the process of re-learning how to walk; I could value doing my best in my job as a trainer, as a husband and friend, as a creative thinker, as a positive and empathic person, and as an enthusiastic role model. I began to measure success by how much acknowledgement and gratitude I gave to others. If becoming aware of my Being Image paved the way for me to keep wellness in mind, it can do the same for all of us. Therefore, let's reframe our understanding of wellness to include Being Image.

Human beings are so lucky. Our brains can actually transform their structure or function in response to outside causes—and we retain this amazing ability all our lives. Scientists call this phenomenon "neuroplasticity." We can exercise neuroplasticity to reframe our understanding of wellness. Reframing is a vitally important first step to change our perspective and enhance our wellness.

To start seeing wellness from the perspective of Being Image, first we need to understand humanity's basic needs. According to Professor of Psychology Darcia Narvaez, a basic need "is a need that, when not met, leads to worse outcomes for physical, mental or social health and well-being."[3]

The classic work on basic needs comes from Abraham Maslow.[4] From his research Maslow identified five stages of needs human beings must satisfy, starting with the first and lowest in his hierarchy: basic life needs such as air, food, drink, shelter, warmth, sex, and sleep. Once these biological needs are satisfied, we can focus on the second-stage needs of protection and security. The third-stage needs in the hierarchy include belongingness and love needs (family, affection, relationships, work group, etc.). The fourth stage pertains to esteem needs such as achievement, status, responsibility, and reputation. The fifth and final level focuses on self-actualization, which includes needs of personal growth and fulfillment.

We agree with Professor Narvaez who suggests that some additional needs should be added to Maslow's hierarchy. She suggests adding "intersubjectivity with others, reciprocity, and coregulation of all our physiological and psychological systems."[5] Translation: this is the very principle of mirroring, empathic co-creation that Being Image is based on. For more of the fascinating science behind this, see "How We Are I-Other" in the Appendix.

Here is an important question that we need to ask as part of the reframing process. How can we receive our being from someone without rivalry or comparison? The answer to this question lies in the difference between *need* and *desire*.

One distinction is that our needs can be satisfied as a result of *having*—to *do* good for ourselves. We can have our needs met for physiological life, safety, belonging, esteem, self-actualization, and reciprocity with another.

Desire—our innate urge to connect with a loving other—is a matter of *being*. It is openness to co-creation wherein we maximize our potential to *be* good. A new way of being leads us to a new way of behaving with wellness for ourselves and for each other. We are made to imitate and connect with others. When we connect in love, we know we are loved and we love in return.

The point here is, since we are imitative by nature, we must be careful about who we imitate. Imitation constitutes openness to others that is intrinsically good but it only leads to wellness when we imitate non-rivalrous others. We need to imitate those who are able to be advocates, contributing to our well-being. In other words we require others to be *towards* us, for our good, and not *against* us to our detriment.

Most of us realize that our environment affects us. Let's take a look at a little social ecology—the study of people in an environment, and the ways people and environment interact—to learn more about how we influence each other.

The socio-ecological model gives us a big-picture framework for examining factors that influence our wellness. After all, our individual behavior is determined to a large extent by social environment, that is, by community norms and values, regulations, and policies.[6] If a community as a whole shares barriers to healthy behaviors, and if these barriers can be lowered or removed, then individual change immediately becomes more achievable and sustainable.

In the Socio-Ecological model, there are five levels that influence wellness:[7] The **individual level** identifies the knowledge, beliefs, attitudes, and skills that the individual brings to wellness. Some of these factors include age, education, and lifestyle. The **interpersonal level** examines the family members, friends, and social networks that may impact wellness. Some of these factors include attachment patterns and role models. The **organizational level** examines the establishments and social institutions where change can happen. These include schools, workplaces, and neighborhoods. The **community level** explores the relationships among organizations and seeks to identify the characteristics of these relationships that are associated with wellness or that serve as barriers to wellness. The **public policy level** looks at the national, state, and local laws that help create a climate in which wellness is either encouraged or inhibited.

Each of us lives within all five levels of the socio-ecological model. These levels are the places where change can happen. As attitudes, beliefs, knowledge, and skills travel with the individual through the levels, each level is interwoven, and each affects the others. To highlight the crucibles we all go through in life, here is more of Andrew's story. It shows how he reframed wellness after his accident. If he can put wellness in action, so can you.

More of Andrew's Story

My accident shoved me down to the two lowest-stages of Maslow's needs, those of biological/physical homeostasis[i] and safety. I had to learn how to maneuver my body without a left foot. To begin relearning how to walk, I focused on educating myself about Symes amputations and foot prostheses.

When I received my new carbon-fiber foot, I first felt overwhelmingly disappointed. The foot was uncomfortable. The socket seemed bulky. The bulbous ankle area looked ugly. I knew I needed a positive focus, rather than obsessing about my discomfort and disappointment.

Before my accident, as part of my job I had developed physical fitness tests for corrections officers at the Bernalillo County Metropolitan Detention Center. Now I committed to passing those requirements with only one foot. Of the six fitness tests required of all corrections officers, the 1.5-mile run promised to be the most difficult for me. The cut-off time

---

[i] Homeostasis is our body's attempt to maintain internal biological and chemical stability.

for the run was nineteen minutes and fifty-three seconds. I hadn't run in four months. I couldn't even walk without pain, much less jog for a mile and a half on a track made of pavement and hard gravel. While I did not know where my effort would end, I knew what my first step must be. I just had to begin.

Since I couldn't run, I walked. Since I couldn't walk for a full mile and a half, I walked half of that. After a couple of months I employed light interval training alternating between walking fast and jogging. Three months later I timed half the course at ten minutes. Assuming I could maintain pace, it would take me twenty minutes to complete the full course.

I then made a deal with myself. I would segue into the full course if I could complete the first half in nine minutes flat. Since my residual limb still couldn't withstand a consistent jog, I continued with my interpretation of Fartlek training, alternating walking fast with jogging.[ii] The effort required continuous pain management.

Almost a year from the time I became an amputee, I joined a group of twenty cadets to run the 1.5-mile test. Understanding the importance of interconnection, I focused my attention on a cadet who was jogging at a pace I knew was well under the cut-off time. I would jog past her and then walk. When she cruised by me, I would again jog and pass her. I passed the test in seventeen minutes and forty-five seconds. She also passed the test. Together our energies had fueled each other. We had co-created two people who had the physical capacity required of corrections officers in a detention center.

The key that opened the door to my healing journey was reframing my accident. I began to embrace my beingness instead of wallowing in the guilt of recklessness. As I experienced love within the physical trauma of a foot amputation, my wishes to send that love back out into the world increased. Finding the key to wellness within what was actual, real, and true became a core concept for my teachings on wellness.

[ii] "Fartlek" means "speed play" in Swedish. It is a method that blends continuous training with interval training. The intensity and/or speed of the training vary according to the athlete's needs. Most Fartlek sessions last a minimum of forty-five minutes. They can include both aerobic walking and also anaerobic sprinting.

Finally, my forced solitude while recovering at home—the "slowing down" that Cousin Ricky recommended—brought me a felt understanding of peace. That felt peace improved my self-esteem. I came to accept my coping mechanisms as dynamic parts of my desire to *be* good so that in relationship I could bring contentment to others, experience contentment with others, and sustain the goodness of both myself and others.[8] This was in stark contrast to my former efforts to do good for myself, whereas the wellness of others was secondary. Efforts to do good had blocked me from the joy of co-creation.

My desire to be good, however, opened me to experiencing first-hand the interdependence of physical and emotional health. I knew the reality of how much we need one another; we are inter-beings—we begin in union. Throughout my healing journey I kept the wellness of others in my consciousness.

Yes, I had Wellness in Mind.

Now that you've had a chance to understand Being Image, we offer a thought-provoking activity called "My Being Image Blueprint" located in the Wellness in Mind Activities section. Before you go there, here is a blueprint of Andrew's values, vision and mission, just to give you some ideas and context.

Andrew's Values

I value family and the four most important people in my life are my wife because she is the love of my life, my daughter and son because they are extensions of my care, and my father because he is the biological connection to my upbringing.

Andrew's Vision

I am a provider who protects a healthy family that is physically and emotionally safe through a hearty, spirited, and grounded faith. I carry happiness for self, others, and all with whom I come into contact and maintain health through balanced movement, play, and nourishment.

Andrew's Mission

My mission is to cultivate family, faith, happiness, and health, and to give away my nourishing wellness energy to others.

Andrew's mission statement is his Being Image of himself at his very best with the ones he loves most. Establishing values, envisioning success, and declaring a mission provides three important first steps to well-being: an altruistic basis for what he does, a mental picture of what he wants, and a targeted focus on the daily finish line of life.

Your Being Image blueprint is the basis for any wellness activities you undertake, so take some time to fill it out now, and be as honest with yourself as you can.

Chapter 2

Move It!

I move, therefore I am.

—Haruki Murakami

No matter how much of a couch potato you may be, here is a fact that will inspire: our bodies want to move. They are not only designed to move, they need to move in order to remain in balance. Many of us read the word "exercise" and instantly summon visions of grueling workouts and endless hours on a treadmill like a hamster on a wheel. But movement can be a pleasure, not a chore! We want to give you some keys to joyful movement, but first we need to help you make peace with the body you were given.

The "ideal" female model has, until recently, been painfully, unhealthily thin with impossibly long legs (often photo shopped to appear that way) with cheekbones sharp enough to cut a carrot. The "ultimate" male body image is buff and toned, without an ounce of fat anywhere, with abs on demand. These images have caused untold harm, especially to many adolescents who develop eating disorders in the quest for thinness, or who injure themselves trying to attain the impossible.

We need to move beyond simplistic "fat or thin" distinctions, and learn to value the benefits movement offers us, no matter what shape we're in. Physical fitness is the first dimension of wellness, and it becomes important—and liberating—to accept our body as our unique gift, regardless of body type. There are three of them.

> ## SOMATOTYPES
>
> "Somatotype" is the scientific term for a particular build or type of body based on physical characteristics. Here are the three basic somatotypes:
> Endomorph – a person whose body has a husky build and a prominent abdomen.
> Ectomorph – someone who is tall with long, lean limbs.
> Mesomorph – an individual with a stocky, muscular body.

Most of us are a blend of somatotypes. For example, at first glance professional bodybuilders look like heavily-muscled mesomorphs, but close examination of their often-thin joints reveal ectomorph traits. The slender linkages of this meso-ecto combination actually make muscles appear bigger. The point being we are all formed in special ways. While only a select few are born to be pro athletes, we are all built to move!

Whatever the somatotype we've been given, we can learn to honor it. After all, our bodies are an important part of our Being Image. The body is a powerful expression of who we are. It allows us to experience the world through movement, and we can be healthy with the unique form we have.

Before we can understand our body's need for and response to exercise, we have to look at the concept of homeostasis. French physiologist Claude Bernard came up with the term, and American physiologist Walter Bradford Cannon popularized it in 1932. "Homeostasis" is defined as the tendency of biological systems to maintain relatively constant conditions in their internal environments while continuously interacting with and adjusting to changes originating within or outside their systems.[1]

Simply put, the body is constantly balancing itself. It is through homeostatic mechanisms that body temperature is kept within normal range, osmotic pressure of the blood and its hydrogen ion concentration (pH) is kept within strict limits, nutrients are supplied to cells as needed and waste products are removed before they accumulate and reach toxic levels. These are just a few examples of the thousands of homeostatic control systems within our body. Some of these systems operate within our cells and others operate within groups of cells, coordinating complex interrelationships among our various organs. The body is amazingly effective, constantly protecting our health with its ceaseless balancing acts.

Balance is a basic need of our Being Image. As Walter Bradford Cannon said in *The Wisdom of the Body*, "The word [homeostasis] does not imply something set and immobile, a stagnation. It means a condition—a condition which may vary, but which is relatively constant." In other words balance is not flatline; it means movement.

When we have a good relationship with our bodies, we have fitness, and homeostasis supports and sustains fitness. But what is physical fitness, exactly? Here's a handy definition: *Physical fitness is the body's ability to move, play, and work with proficiency.*

Okay. Now ask yourself the following questions based around your fitness: Can I move with proficiency? Am I injury free? Do I truly enjoy myself when exercising? Am I healthy as measured by medical standards? Can my body resist disease? Can I perform strenuous physical exertion to handle an emergency situation? If the answer was "no" to any of these, take heart: this book is designed to help.

Exercise is defined as any activity requiring physical effort that is carried out to sustain or improve health and fitness. To link this definition to Being Image, we would add that exercise should also be fun! As we turn our thoughts to crafting a well-rounded exercise plan for greater physical fitness, we need to be aware of four important components:[2]

FOUR COMPONENTS OF EXERCISE

1. **Cardiorespiratory Fitness**. Aerobic exercise consists of rhythmic, continuous, and repetitive movements with major muscle groups. It maintains and improves cardiovascular fitness so that our body can adequately deliver oxygen to its working muscles, which need oxygen to convert calories into energy. Without enough oxygen, muscles and body become fatigued and subject to illness and injury.

2. **Muscle Strength**. Muscle strength is defined as absolute strength, which is tested by a one-repetition maximum lift of weight. Calisthenics, free weights, or machines can be a means of maintaining or increasing muscle strength. It is important to include exercises for every major muscle group, including the muscles of arms, chest, back, stomach, hips, and legs. The American Council on Exercise (ACE) recommends starting with a weight that is comfortable to handle and performing eight repetitions. For greater strength conditioning, add more weight and/or more repetitions (in sets of eight to twelve) when the exercise becomes easy.

3. **Muscle Endurance**. Muscle endurance is the ability of muscles to perform consistently for prolonged periods of time. Similar to muscle strength, calisthenics, free weights, or machines can be a means of maintaining or increasing endurance and it is important to include exercises for every major muscle group. ACE recommends starting with a weight that is comfortable to handle and performing eight repetitions. Gradually add more repetitions until twelve is reached. Increase weight when the twelve repetitions become easy.

4. **Flexibility**. Flexibility is maintained by stretching, which can be either dynamic or static. *Dynamic Stretching* is stretching body parts through movement and should be performed as a pre-workout warm-up to transition our body from rest to activity. *Static Stretching* is stretching performed without movement that is generally performed after a workout when our muscles are warm. Slowly and easily hold the muscle being stretched at the furthest range of motion for twenty to thirty seconds while breathing deeply. Stretching should be relaxing and should not hurt.

In addition to the four components of exercise, we need to be aware of three exercise stages as we prepare to strategize a physical fitness plan. To avoid injuring yourself and to maximize your enjoyment, it is vital to understand these stages, perform them in order, and be mindful of time limits within each stage.

THREE STAGES OF EXERCISE

1. **Warm-up Stage**. Lasting five to ten minutes, warming up moves our body from rest to activity. The warm-up may include:
   - Exercise activity at a low intensity (walking at a very slow pace, for example)
   - Static stretching (good for those of us who feel out of shape)
   - Active isolated stretching (good for someone in good condition)
   - Dynamic and ballistic stretching (good for a performance athlete)

2. **Conditioning Stage**. This follows the warm-up. For best results, the American College of Sports Medicine recommends the FITT Principle, a handy acronym that stands for Frequency, Intensity, Type and Time:

   Frequency – The Centers for Disease Control and Prevention (CDC) recommends a minimum for adults of 150 minutes of moderate-intensity aerobic activity (brisk walking) every week and muscle-strengthening activities on two or more days a week.

   Intensity – Should challenge our body but not be so difficult that it injures or discourages us.

   Type – Refers to the kind of exercise we choose. For example, with cardiovascular training the exercise should be continuous in nature and make use of large muscle groups as when we run, walk, swim, or cycle. Strength training would involve lifting free or machine weights.

   Time – Refers to how long we exercise. With regard to cardiovascular training, people with lower fitness levels should maintain cardiovascular endurance activity for twenty to thirty minutes. The muscular strength and endurance training range is between twenty to thirty minutes up to but not exceeding forty-five to sixty minutes. The entire conditioning stage of exercise— encompassing the FITT Principle—consists of thirty to forty minutes of continuous exercise or ten-minute increments to equal thirty to forty minutes through the day.

3. **Cool-down Stage**. This last stage allows our body to recover from the conditioning phase. Cooling down does not mean sitting down! In fact we should not stand still, sit, or lie down right after exercise or we might feel dizzy, become lightheaded, or have palpitations.
   - Slowly decrease the intensity of the activity.
   - Perform the stretching and low intensity exercises from the warm-up phase.

With our Being Image blueprint from Chapter 1 in hand, we can now begin to reframe our concept of exercise, seeing it through the lens of enjoyment rather than duty, of fun rather than pain—in other words, placing physical fitness in the frame of our Being Image. After all, if being happy is part of wellness, how can we expect to feel happy doing things that feel like a chore?

As if we didn't know this already, the National Weight Control Registry—the largest investigation of long-term successful weight loss maintenance—has shown that exercise and diet are keys to losing weight. But this book has larger wellness goals than simple weight loss. Instead, we endorse play and proper fuel as important Being Image goals.

It's easy to make pleasure a goal for any physical fitness activity. All it takes are these eight keys that help us experience joy:[3] The activity (1) can be completed; (2) engages concentration; (3) has clear goals; (4) provides immediate feedback; (5) consists of a deep but effortless involvement that removes from awareness the worries and frustrations of everyday life; (6) allows a sense of control over our actions; (7) makes concern for self disappear as sense of beingness emerges; and (8) sense of time is altered (hours seem like minutes).

Here is Andrew's account of how adjusting his exercise routine led to experiencing all eight keys:

Reviving an Enjoyable Exercise Routine

After my accident, my journey to wellness continued to revolve around adaptation to my injuries. I did not have a normal shoulder, I had a skinny stump for a lower leg, and I constantly dealt with phantom pain (perceived pain amputees commonly feel). As a result, I quickly became an expert in postural awareness, back and spine exercises, myofascial release (massage with a foam roll), and even became an active stretcher (a task I dreaded in the past).

As I progressed physically, I decided to start something I used to do regularly with friend and mentor Art De La Cruz: run the ditch banks by the river behind his house. I began the old routine on a crisp fall morning by enjoying a short traffic-less drive to Art's house. Upon arrival, I gently warmed up with dynamic stretches of my lower back and trunk. During the jog with Art, we enjoyed light conversation and before I knew it, we had completed the run. After some static stretching (and a cup of coffee) I drove back home feeling my Being Image enhanced by a completed task.

At home I evaluated our activity according to the eight major keys to enjoyment:

> *Task can be completed*: The jog took less than forty-five minutes.
> *Task engages concentration*: We focused on breathing and running form.
> *Clear goals*: We completed the course without stopping.
> *Immediate feedback*: The gentle cardiovascular endurance exercise induced a light sweat, increased blood flow, detoxified our bodies through perspiration, and provided physiological proof of immediate success through the release of pleasurable hormones.
> *Removes worries*: Our minds were absorbed in the sounds of nature and fellowship.
> *Control over actions*: We completed the three stages of exercise.
> *Sense of beingness*: Our Being Images were enhanced by maintaining healthy and functional bodies that uphold our life values.
> *Sense of time altered*: Our jogging cadence, the beautiful views of nature, and casual chitchat made the run seem timeless.
> That's time well spent!

Andrew's example shows us how easy it can be to turn a routine exercise regimen into a fun personal movement activity. Here are some other suggestions to maximize activities of daily living: Walk with a coworker during lunch break or with a friend (or your pet) in the evening. Take advantage of wellness incentive campaigns if they are employer-provided. Choose a form of exercise through hobbies and leisure activities, and view home projects as opportunities to hone both fine and gross motor skills.

If you're motivated to do more (or less) with your movement program, assess how the three exercise stages contribute to your feeling of well-being by taking this quick Movement Quiz: Does each stage recharge my beingness? How are my limitations challenged? How does my mind feel after the workout? Did I escape reality/time? Does my body feel replenished?

The traditional model of exercise that identifies the four components of fitness is a safe way for beginners or folks coming off a long layoff from exercise to start a joyful journey of movement and play. However, over the last twenty-five years contemporary fitness models have expanded to address more than these four basics. Exciting news is coming out of the fitness industry every day. Now, physical fitness is commonly viewed as a continuum of function, health, fitness, and performance. Certified personal trainers routinely address psychological health-behavior changes, postural stability, kinetic chain mobility, movement efficiency, core conditioning, balance, cardiorespiratory fitness (aerobic and anaerobic), metabolic markers (ventilatory thresholds), and sports performance measures such as agility, coordination and reactivity, speed, and power. The list goes on and on. If you decide to scout for a personal trainer to coach and support you in your fitness goals, we recommend you take a look at "Professional Credentials" in the Appendix.

It's good to remember that we are meant to be moving beings and activities of daily living can become the physical fitness stimulus of life-long Being Image goals. After all, a healthy beingness creates positive energy and flows out to touch others. The more energy we have, the more lives we touch.

Chapter 3

No More Starving! Fuel Yourself with Food and Love

There's this relentless and powerful marketing of foods, you're basically taught that you can eat everywhere, you can eat ever hour of the day, and that there's something gloriously wonderful about eating foods that are high in sugar, fat and salt.

—Kelly Brownell, Ph.D., Director
Rudd Center for Food Policy and Obesity
Yale University

We know high sugar consumption is related to type 2 diabetes, high salt ingestion affects blood pressure, and high saturated fat intake is connected to coronary heart disease. These are leading causes of death and touch the lives of almost 120 million Americans. The issue of nutrition becomes even more complicated when we realize true nourishment comes from psychological nurturing as well as from physiological nourishment.

Remember Kelly's story from Chapter 1? Even if we were never given the emotional nurturing we needed, we can learn how to fill ourselves with love and nourishment. Like Kelly, we can create new neural connections in our brains so we can thrive rather than simply survive.

Whereas Kelly was literally starving herself, many of us overeat unhealthy foods in a misguided attempt to feel nourished, full, and loved. Every time we succumb to advertising's siren song to eat the salt, sugar, and fat packed into foods on every grocery store shelf, especially in the form of packaged foods, we diminish our being. But when we discover the true nourishment found in meaningful relationships and in nutrient-packed whole foods, the negative cycle that can lead to disease is broken and we begin to truly feast on life.

Here's an important question: How can I stop starving myself (which often includes stuffing the body with empty-calorie foods in an attempt to feel fed) and begin feasting on all that life offers?

Five allies hold the answer.

Boost critical thinking skills – Why don't ads showcase the spectacular pleasures of whole foods or highlight the abundant options for natural nourishment? Simple, it's because the big corporations won't profit. Yes, agribusiness is catching on that there is money to be made in the health-food market, but it often involves the misleading use of words like "healthy" and "all-natural," when the products are actually anything but. The buyer must definitely beware!

Critical thinking begins with awareness of just how big the business of weight loss is. *U.S. Weight Loss & Diet Control Market*[1] claims that the total weight loss market in the United States tops $60 billion. Commercial weight loss chains promise instant gratification with diet drugs, diet pills, meal replacements, diet programs, diet websites, diet apps, home delivery services and more. Compounding the influence of the weight loss business is our nation's overproduction of certain foods (corn, beef, and dairy are heavily subsidized by our government) and the fortification and enrichment of products by artificially increasing micronutrients[iii] or by

---

[iii] Micronutrients are vitamins and minerals that are essential for and promote cellular function. Macronutrients are substances our bodies need in relatively large amounts (proteins, carbohydrates, and fats). Macronutrients provide calories for energy; they also perform other functions such as tissue repair, immune system functioning, hormone and enzyme production, and maintenance of lean muscle mass and tone.

replacing original nutrients removed or destroyed through processing—all in the name of increasing product shelf life.

In a perfect world, we could simply follow government food guidelines to improve our nutrition. But we don't live in a perfect world. Government watchdogs are challenged to adequately govern the food industry because we are targets of relentless marketing that messes with our minds, making us think we must have what we don't need and sidetracking us from buying what we most need. In the end, it's up to Joe Public to think critically about target marketing and understand how food processing and food promotion impact nutrition.

Beyond food labels, we can learn a lot from the descriptions on packaged goods. *Refined* involves the removal of impurities or unwanted elements from a substance, such as refined sugar. *Fortified* means to increase essential micronutrients such as vitamins and minerals in processed food. Food products can also be fortified with nutrients that weren't in the original food before processing. *Enriched* is synonymous with fortification, but also includes the addition of micronutrients that were lost during the processing of the food. You would think all this is a good thing, a means of reducing disease caused by dietary deficiency. But look again.

Food promoters scare people into feeling that we are deficient in something like certain vitamins and minerals, for example. So, rather than buying whole foods naturally rich in micronutrients our bodies can utilize, we choose refined products, fortified and enriched with chemical micronutrients that our bodies may not even be able to absorb properly.

Minimize the three major ingredients of processed and fast foods – Our fast food nation invests millions of dollars in research and development to create food-like products that reward our brains but that our bodies barely recognize as food. Advertisers seduce us with product claims coupled with visual and auditory stimuli, like television commercials that create artificial thirst for sugary beverages as children aspire to be like their favorite professional athlete. Billions are spent marketing these unhealthy products and branding them into our brains. Much of the actual nutrition is removed and what is left is salted, sugared, and fattened. In fact, many of the ingredients in processed foods are synthetic creations of chemists to reward our brains through "bliss points," "mouth feel," and "allure." A must-read on this subject is Pulitzer Prize recipient Michael Moss's investigatory gem, *Salt Sugar Fat: How the Food Giants Hooked Us*.

The acronym **3SP** is an easy way to keep Wellness in Mind in all your culinary environments. Let's start with the letter 'S'. 3S reminds us to limit salt, sugar, and saturated fat, the primary ingredients of most processed foods proven to be harmful to our health when consumed in excess. 3P induces critical thinking behind product, preparation, and promotion.

What are those 3S ingredients again? Salt, Sugar, and Saturated fat.

Most Americans take in far, far more than the recommended daily allowance for each of these—sometimes as much as three times more per day, most of it in the form of processed, packaged, or fast food. Here are the actual recommended allowances for salt, sugar and saturated fat:

Salt (1,500 mg)[2,3]
Sugar (women: 25 g; men: 37.5 g)[4]
Saturated Fat (20g; Total Fat 65g)

Boost those critical thinking skills by learning to read labels! Here is a simple way to activate critical thinking in the grocery store. When making food choices, remember the 3P's: Product, Preparation and Promotion.

What kind of product am I choosing? Is it real food or a food-like product? What types of preparation did my food go through before arriving on my plate? Is it fresh, live food? If not, how was it cooked? How was it preserved? How long did the product take to get to me? What kind of promotion revolves around my food? Am I paying a premium price for the marketing costs of an inferior product? Am I ignoring nutritional need to feed my wants of entertainment and socialization?

For an important disclaimer, see "The Acronym 3SP, a Note" in the Appendix.

Maximize nutrient-dense foods – We need nutrient-dense foods to replenish and repair micro-damaged cells and to rejuvenate our bodies. So here are a couple of sure-fire strategies for making sure our diets include plenty of them:

First, learn to recognize them. What are nutrient-dense foods? They are natural foods that provide substantial amounts of vitamins, minerals and antioxidants, even when eaten in small amounts. And they contain relatively few calories. A rule of thumb is nutrient-dense foods are whole foods (quinoa and millet, rather than refined white-flour pasta, for example). Another tip is nutrient-dense foods are often naturally colorful. For instance, blackberries, orange squash, and kale are all strongly colored and they all pack a nutritional punch.

Second, enjoy eating them. Just as focusing on pleasure placed physical fitness in the frame of Being Image, we can do the same with eating. Remember that Kelly's nurturing of her heart emotionally and psychologically required the physiological experience of intersubjective resonance—of loving empathy. Likewise, nurturing our bodies requires not only physiological feeding with nutrient-dense foods but also the emotional and psychological experience of enjoyment. Enhance the appeal of your food with alluring preparation techniques and creative presentations.

Keep Good Food Nearby – When you go to the store, buy only the best quality, freshest food you can afford. Refuse to stock up on sugary sodas and greasy chips and invest in your health with lots of vibrant, colorful, delicious whole foods. Better yet, make weekly visits to your local farmer's market or join a CSA (Community Supported Agriculture) and get the freshest food right from the source. Keeping good food nearby also requires an understanding of government watchdogs and target marketing. For some enlightening (and somewhat alarming) information, see "Government Watchdogs" in the Appendix.

Typical weight-loss efforts that focus solely on calorie restriction are doomed to fail, because restrictive dieting is about food limitation and rejection. When we fall off the starvation wagon, so many of us make the negative promise, "I'll never let that happen again" but we do, over and over again. So much negativity! Instead, keeping our Being Image in mind creates a positive mindset. We can make affirming statements like, "Fuel yourself" to seek out delicious fare the human body needs. By eating real food we become viscerally aware of our own response to hunger, appetite, and satiety.

VISCERAL AWARENESS

Hunger is our biological signal to nourish our bodies. Hunger should be embraced and respected as a life-giving communication from our body. Listening to our body and taking the time to care for its needs are critical steps in loving and caring for ourselves. Hunger signs vary from person to person, but they arrive to let us know that our stomachs are empty, most commonly through signals like growling stomach, light-headedness, headache, irritability, and lack of concentration.

Appetite is based on stimuli such as our social situation, food availability, or just plain habit. Sometimes we do not know why our appetite controls our eating. Unlike hunger, which is primarily a biological phenomenon, appetite is primarily a psychological phenomenon.

Satiety is a complex interaction of both biological and psychological factors and is defined by the quality or state of being gratified to the point of satisfaction.

There is one biological factor: *Sensory-specific satiety*.[5] Sensory-specific satiety is declining satisfaction generated by the consumption of a certain type of food. Appetite can be renewed by exposure to a new flavor. So, even if we fill up at a buffet on one specific food, we may feel hungry again when we see another type of fare.

There are two psychological factors: *Conditioned satiety* refers to appetite being suppressed by the effects of eating such as bloating, which occurs when a food with a given flavor is eaten on a partly full stomach. *Alimentary alliesthesia* refers to a person's internal state that elicits a pleasant or unpleasant reaction to food. Forms of alliesthesia are thermic (hot and cold), olfactory (smell), gustatory (taste), olfacto-gustatory (smell-taste), visual/optic (sight) and auditory (hearing). Each of these forms of alliesthesia exists in two opposite tendencies: negative alliesthesia that transforms the sensation from pleasure to displeasure and positive alliesthesia that transforms the sensation from displeasure to pleasure.

The point is both biological and psychological factors affect hunger, appetite, and satiety. They change with changes in lifestyle, environment, season, age, and health. When synthesized into our daily lives, the components of our visceral awareness (hunger, appetite, and satiety) enhance our beingness by bringing us into the fullness of health.

Andrew enhanced his understanding of visceral awareness in 2007. Here is his personal story:

Two Simple Rules to Gaining Satisfaction

When I served on the New Mexico Healthier Weight Council, Dr. Brenda Wolfe, Ph.D. and Dr. Duane Ross, M.D. presented a one-day workshop entitled "Foundation of Weight Control," based on visceral awareness techniques developed by Linda Craighead, Ph.D. The workshop began at eight in the morning with Dr. Wolfe asking participants why they had signed up for the workshop. Their answers came spewing out in the form of negative labeling. The first responder said, "I'm here because I eat like a pig. The reason I weigh 10,000 pounds is because I just can't keep my mouth shut and I want to know what your secret is." The other attendees gave similar responses. Their collective energy was one of self-hatred, anger, and desperation. They really needed some intrasubjective resonance with their own bodies—like the resonance Kelly discovered with Dr. Sally.

Dr. Wolfe announced that she planned on serving lunch at one in the afternoon to ensure everyone was truly tummy-growl hungry. Indeed, I was ravenous by the time the food arrived. I sat down to a turkey wrap with a small pasta salad, fully intent on cleaning up at least two plates according to the habit of over-eating that I formed as a teenager and continued into adulthood.

Dr. Wolfe slammed the brakes on my plans, giving explicit instructions for attuning to our visceral awareness. She gave us two simple guidelines. First rule: When food is in your mouth, keep your hands empty. We were instructed to put a small bite in our mouth and put down our fork. We were to taste the food fully by completely chewing the bite into a liquid. Once we swallowed the bite, we could take our fork and get another bite. Second rule: Conduct a body inventory after every three bites. This strategy included a handout we had been given with a circle on it to represent our stomach. The body inventory included the following introspective questions: How do your extremities feel? How does your mind feel? How does your chest cavity feel? How does your stomach feel?

Every three bites, we had to draw a line through our "stomach" to indicate our changing level of satiety. While I had to struggle mightily on the first bite to keep my nervous hands empty, I stuck to the rules just to see where they would take me. In the end, I could only muster enough hunger to take twenty-one bites of food before I was satisfied. Twenty-one small bites of food! Amazing!

What I anticipated would be a plate-clearing pig-at-the-trough spectacle had turned into a respectful and very enjoyable meal that ended with a third of the turkey wrap and small bit of pasta salad remaining on my plate. In just one very controlled setting with two simple rules to follow, I discovered that food tastes better when taken in smaller bites.

Smaller bites and chewing thoroughly allows for the enzyme amylase to break down food into liquid. I had allowed the time necessary to feel my levels of satiety viscerally and assess each one cognitively. My stomach did not feel overwhelmed. I ate until satisfied and left on my plate an amount that would have stuffed me. I allowed my hunger pangs to subside by eating completely and with grace, allowing my body not only to reach satiety, but also to give my brain ample time to receive the important signal of satisfaction.

To this day, I practice visceral awareness with some added flare. Whenever I get a craving, I ask myself: What sounds the most appealing? What looks the most appealing? What taste am I craving (sweet, salty, or sour)? What texture feels good (crunchy, crispy, or creamy)? What smells appetizing? Natural foods bring great pleasure and have the benefit of satisfying all my five senses. Precision in behavior begins with enjoyment. This thoroughness of enjoyment slows the eating process down even more so I eat until satisfied and leave 'stuffed' on the plate!

Remember the following helpful hints: Avoid using your first brain (mind) to control your second brain (stomach); eyes are bigger than stomachs and can generate false hunger; differentiate between emotional hunger and biological hunger; love and belonging—associative intersubjective hunger—need satisfying; under the influence lowers inhibitions.

Amplify awareness by asking the following questions: Am I eating enough live produce for optimal health? Do I attempt to enjoy healthful foods that feed my beingness or am I substituting food for love and belonging?

Am I preparing food for the renewal of life? To help you come to a place of pleasure and wellness around eating, there is a "Healthy-Eating Satisfaction Survey" in the Wellness in Mind Activities section that you can use.

Make Culinary Connections – For many of us, eating is our default activity when we are lonely, bored, or stressed, and the foods we choose at such times are unlikely to be the healthiest. Instead of eating something beyond your wellness priorities why not connect with someone such as phoning a friend, suggesting a walk-and-talk, going to a pick-your-own farm and filling a basket with fresh strawberries and apples, or cooking a meal and sharing it with one another. Why not go to the root of what we need and connect with a family member, sign up for an interesting workshop, or take a fifteen-minute meditation or relaxation break instead of reaching for the gallon of ice cream? We need to use our self-loving critical skills to alert us when the greed-driven marketing of unhealthy food is misleading us. As Kelly's story has shown, love and food go hand in hand for all of us: we need both forms of nourishment. The gathering, preparing, and cooking of food is a time-honored way to connect with others. Love makes food taste better, and the experience of a meal shared with a dear one nourishes us body and soul.

FUEL AND NOURISH

You can eat plentifully and nourish your body to replenish, rejuvenate and heal. Operate at optimal levels by applying the following general principles:

Plan, prepare, and pack for the daily journey of wellness.

Consider the effects that the food and drink you
choose have on mind, body and spirit.

Honor meal preparation as a creative experience.

Be present with your meal by preventing distraction.

Show gratitude for nourishment; not all human beings enjoy the honor.

Savor each taste through all your senses until hunger is satisfied.

Remember "feeling satisfied" is the most accurate form of moderation.

Be alert: Our regulator eating signals are conveyed through whispers.

Eat until satisfied—leave stuffed on the plate!

Becoming and staying a healthy weight is a choice between enjoyment and suffering. They are mutually exclusive. As actor Morgan Freeman's character declares in the movie *Shawshank Redemption,* "Get busy living or get busy dying." The choice is ours.

PART II

INTROSPECTION: KNOW YOURSELF TO ENHANCE YOUR WELLNESS HABITS

This section is an empowering look at the negative habits that can often derail us and prevent us from making positive wellness changes. Once you become aware of the places where you get stuck, we can show you how to move past them into true wellness.

Chapter 4

Wellness: It's All in Your Head

> The greatest discovery of my generation is that human beings can alter their lives by altering their attitudes of mind.
>
> —William James (1842-1910)

How many times have you or someone you know asked one or more of the following questions? Why can't I stay with an exercise program? Why can't I lose weight? Why can't I start? Why can't I quit? Why aren't my actions consistent with my wellness goals? Why aren't my core values always lived out in what I do?

The secrets to gaining health from the inside out reside in our minds. If our ability to move toward wellness was only determined by our perception of external reality, we'd all be onboard the wellness train. But the truth is that our non-conscious internal reality also affects our perception.[1]

We've already talked about the amazing phenomenon of neural plasticity, which means we can change our brains. But the same phenomenon also means that our brains are inscribed with our life experiences. Some of those inscriptions can rearrange themselves. They can, in effect, communicate among themselves and produce new inscriptions. But those new inscriptions are no longer in direct connection with the initial perception. They can escape our conscious awareness. In fact, some are completely inaccessible to awareness;[2] yet they still affect the attitudes of our mind.

It is important to bring these unconscious inscriptions to mind. Those inscriptions that are non-conscious from the outset were most probably laid down in our brain during the first months of life where the right hemisphere—which processes non-verbal intersubjective communications, emotional regulation, and body awareness—is growing more rapidly than the left.[3, 4] In addition to being laid down in our right hemisphere, non-conscious inscriptions may also be laid down in part of our brain called the amygdala,[5] which processes emotional images and beliefs that affect how we perceive reality.

This is significant. It means that William James was right: we can alter our lives by altering the attitudes of our minds. The challenge is to bring our intentions and our actions for wellness into consciousness and synchrony so that we can relate to our Being Image, others, and the world in a well way. To do this, we need to acknowledge things inside our brain that distract us from wellness.

Blind spots, barriers, and burdens are internal predispositions that often distract us from wellness. They arise from a complex interplay of genetic endowment, intersubjective experiences during our formative years, cultural learning, and mental/physiological states. These tendencies can affect our ability to perceive reality clearly and our efforts to bring wellness to our entire being by clouding the frame through which we perceive our wellness reality.

Let's take a closer look at **Blind Spots**. Much like the fictional ostrich with its head in the sand, the inability to see the folly of our actions clearly weakens our ability to make solid wellness decisions. Exercise and diet blind spots can manifest in three different unhealthy behavior patterns:

Unhealthy Coping Mechanisms are maladaptive behaviors applied as wrong solutions to problems, such as overeating to soothe oneself when experiencing stress rather than addressing the stress.

Dissociative Thinking is an inability to connect the dots between unhealthy behaviors and their consequences, such as rationalizing a sugar-and-fat-laden dessert as just reward for hard work in a high power job.

Compensatory Behaviors are actions such as giving to assuage feelings such as guilt, shame, and disappointment instead of giving from the goodness of one's heart. Attempts to soften painful feelings about unwanted behaviors rather than addressing the source problems that caused them can leave us in discord.

All three of these blind spots affect accuracy in thought. Much like the person whose only life-tool is a hammer, these bad habits can become ingrained as our automatic nail-biting reactions to life.

Barriers to gaining health are attitudes and beliefs that do not support wellness, acting like walls that prevent us from taking in new information and living in the present.

Barriers can manifest themselves in three ways:

Cognitive Inertia is "the tendency for beliefs or sets of beliefs to endure once formed...cognitive inertia refers to the human inclination to rely on familiar assumptions and a reluctance and/or inability to revise those assumptions, even when the evidence supporting them no longer exists or when other evidence would question their accuracy."[6]

Cognitive Distortions are thoughts that convince us that something is true when it isn't actually factual. David Burns[7] identifies the most prevalent distortions:

> All-or-Nothing Thinking – Looking at things in black and white terms such as attacking our fitness program like a Navy Seal or not participating in a fitness program at all
>
> Overgeneralization – Viewing a negative event as a continual pattern of defeat
>
> Negative Filtering – Dwelling on the negatives and ignoring the positives
>
> Jumping to Conclusions – Assuming others see us in a diminished light with no basis in reality; erroneously predicting that our wellness efforts will end in failure
>
> Magnification or Minimization – Blowing setbacks out of proportion or diminishing positive actions; discounting our consistent workout attendance because it wasn't intense enough

> Emotional Reasoning – Feeling like a failure establishes failurehood: "I don't feel I can succeed in wellness efforts, so I won't try."
>
> "Should" or Catastrophe Statements – Demanding that oneself or others should, shouldn't, must, ought to, or have to be something
>
> Labeling – Calling oneself or others unsavory names (lazy slug, fat pig, etc.)
>
> Personalization and Blame – Blaming oneself or others inappropriately

America's less-than thinking continues as we chase the magic pills, short-cut elixirs and silver bullets of the exercise and diet industry. Cognitive distortions are the negative feedback loops that chain our internal dialog to the proverbial hamster wheel.

Body Image Focus creates I-It (rather than I-Other) relationships and highlights the faults of self and other. This fuels overly competitive relationships that hinder us from developing our Being Image.

As we diminish the confidence necessary to defeat temptation, our erroneous attitudes and beliefs can block efforts to prepare and take action for change toward health and wellness. This brings us to the third group of internal dispositions.

Burdens are characterized as the thousand-pound gorilla or the overabundant monkeys we carry on our backs. They consist of real and perceived stressors we spend so much time towing around that we end up missing opportunities to enhance our wellness. These could be childhood memories good and bad, behavior that conflicts with our values, and/or negative emotions such as worry. They could also include conflict at home or in the workplace, as well as fear-based attachments.

Burdens that weigh us down can manifest in three areas:

Unrealistic Expectations create personal fitness plans that seem never to produce the desired body-image results we had in mind, such as an overly intense exercise program or extreme diet.

Unresolved Conflict results in lugging around negative intrapersonal and interpersonal emotions that breed anger, fear, frustration, guilt, and shame. These emotions prevent the peace and clarity required for healthy behavior change.

Unrealized Beingness is living in fear-based attachment patterns and establishing fear-based relationships with new people one meets and not realizing who one is created to be—a loving and encouraging person for ourself and for others.

The work of wellness requires us to address our blind spots, barriers, and burdens to enlarge the frame of our wellness perspective through intersubjective truth.[8] This work is a lifelong process of healing wherein we allow ourselves to become curious about ourselves and others. What in our upbringing created us and others as we are? Can we forgive ourselves and others for developing the way we did? Can we look past troublesome behavior to address our own and others' inner beauty? Can we let go of hurt or animosity and respond with love and forgiveness? When we can, we will enhance our total beingness.

When we think about it, we can see that there is a lot of overlap between blind spots, barriers, and burdens, and their complex interrelations can impede even our best efforts to change our lifestyle. Fortunately, we can begin to heal old thought patterns by putting old habits to rest as we build our wellness. We *can* change. And it is the loving security of another that fosters our change. Being is birthed in communion—an outpouring of pure love to gain health from the inside out.

According to the Transtheoretical Model[9,10] of behavioral change, change typically occurs in five stages:

Precontemplation	People are not intending to take action.
Contemplation	People intend to change.
Preparation	People begin to take active steps toward action such as buying a pair of running shoes or signing up with a gym.
Action	People have made specific overt modifications in their lifestyles.
Maintenance	People adhere to new healthful behaviors for at least six months.

These Stages explain when changes in thinking, feeling, and behavior occur.

The Processes of Change are activities that people engage in—both covertly and overtly—to move from one stage of change to the next. According to the Transtheoretical Model, there are ten processes.[11,12]

Early Stage Transitions – Experiential Processes

1. Consciousness Raising means becoming more aware of the causes and effects of problem behaviors and how they can be changed. The three-step process of enhancing Being Image (information, introspection and intersubjectivity) is paramount to increasing awareness.

2. Dramatic Relief involves paying attention to feelings and using emotional experiences to take appropriate action. Reframing our victories in life can move us emotionally to take healthy action. Mobilizing mentors provides the support team for success.

3. Environmental Reevaluation refers to how a particular behavior affects the surrounding social milieu. Consistently choosing environments that are illuminating to beingness enhances the wellness of all. And choosing how to experience and respond to our surroundings can help keep everyone's wellness aspirations in the forefront.

4. Social Liberation requires systems support that can expand the opportunities for people to change their behavior. (You'll read more about systems in Chapter 8.) These include taking stock of ever increasing ways to move, play, fuel, relax, and enjoy life with like-minded advocates.

5. Self-reevaluation means re-assessing one's Being Image by one or more techniques such as viewing our self as a protector of life values for self or others or finding healthy role models.

Later Stage Transitions – Behavioral Processes

6. Stimulus Control refers to ways of supporting change and reducing risks for relapse. Examples are: avoiding unhealthy stimuli,

environmental re-engineering such as planning parking lots with a two-minute walk to the office, and self-help groups.

7. Helping Relationships maintain behavioral change by providing trust and acceptance.

8. Counter Conditioning includes healthy behaviors such as: relaxation to counter stress, assertion to counter peer pressure, nicotine replacement to substitute for cigarettes, and nourishing foods in lieu of processed products. Seek spirit-lifting experiences instead of simply avoiding problem behaviors.

9. Reinforcement Management helps maintain behavioral change by providing processes for success. Contingency contracts, overt and covert reinforcements, positive self-statements, and group recognition can reinforce healthier responses. When stuck in a rut, bolstering "positive self talk" can be a useful reinforcement technique. For example, "Nice workout—I'm glad I called my buddy to play tennis."

10. Self-liberation manifests itself in both the conviction and the commitment to maintain change.

Blind spots, barriers, and burdens are the coping mechanisms we developed to deal with situations in our past but that hinder us from wellness in the present. Uncovering, acknowledging, and properly owning our blind spots liberate us to engage in the processes of change toward wellness. Removing barriers by challenging old beliefs and analyzing assumptions allows us to focus on building new behaviors that strengthen our beingness. Unloading burdens through the acceptance and forgiveness of self and others empowers us with the confidence to search within ourselves to find our reason for being—our Being Image.

Wellness really is all in our heads!

Let's view a real-life example of the difficulties in making change when we do not address our blind spots, barriers, and burdens. See if you can identify the three B's expressed in Andrew's "Client One" story, whose struggles are representative of millions who battle with exercise and diet.

Client One

It was the first of January, a New Year, and Client One enthusiastically made a resolution to improve his fitness. His plan was like that of many American yo-yo dieters and binge exercisers. He swore off sweets and committed himself to losing ten pounds a month over the next three months. He would accomplish this by jogging on the treadmill for one hour every morning, a task he hated but that had proven helpful for losing weight in the past. He would also avoid friends and co-workers who might tempt him to indulge in food and drinks that he had sworn to avoid.

Things were looking up. He lost twelve pounds in January. As hard as it was both physically and emotionally, he felt great and was proud of his progress. He deserved a reward. Besides, he could use a break from the treadmill—the hour of jogging everyday in January had been hurting his knees. To celebrate the month-long accomplishment, he ventured out on a declared "cheat day".

Back at work, he felt a little lonely and missed socializing with his co-workers. Perhaps he'd hang out a bit more. February continued with Client One skipping workouts and falling into old eating habits. Long story short, Client One's resolution for the New Year came to a screeching halt by the middle of March and the weight he lost returned in spades.

What happened? Client One didn't set viable goals. He should have first obtained a physician's clearance to begin an exercise program. Client One didn't implement a well-rounded plan that formed long-term habits of daily living and that considered personal strengths, weaknesses, opportunities, and threats within his environments.

Did you recognize other faulty efforts? Let's review.

Client One's aggressive exercise program and diet plan did not include the FITT principle nor apply tenets within the three stages of exercise. His fitness routine did not include the four components of fitness and cardiovascular training was one-dimensional. Increased treadmill time was used as punishment for overeating and there was not any support for rest or recovery.

He removed potential advocates from his social circles, failed to address high-stress situations at work, and did not prepare responses to emotional triggers created by social situations with friends and co-workers. The routine lacked enjoyment and disregarded nourishing food and drink consumption. His focus was solely on negative behaviors—disallowing the integration of new fitness habits to settle into a wellness lifestyle.

There's more.

He maintained a destructive body image by losing weight without gaining health and by not creating a response plan for upcoming social events. Most important, he did not have an altruistic path for bringing in relationships to co-create enjoyable experiences. As we can clearly see, Client One's three B's were evident in a plethora of mistakes.

Subsequently, Client One engaged in wellness planning with me and worked diligently to widen his frame of wellness by becoming aware of the blind spots, barriers, and burdens that had undermined his actions. Client One brought clarity to his reality and focused on attaining his wellness goals. He moved through the five Stages of Change by letting go of the discouragement of his failed new year's resolution, becoming aware of and responding to internal predispositions, and by preparing a plan for life-style change whereby he replaced faulty habits of being with reliable healthy ones. Focusing on his Being Image—his intersubjective way of viewing his relationship with wellness—he built a fitness plan that did succeed. He was empowered to prevent relapse by embracing the old adage, "Slow and steady wins the race."

Client One's experience shows all of us what can happen when we become conscious of our three B's and use our beingness to move through the stages of change. If he can do it, so can you!

Chapter 5

Bullseye! Target Well-Being for Life

> [N]ot everything that can be counted counts, and not everything that counts can be counted.
>
> —William Bruce Cameron
> *Informal Sociology*

Now we can begin to apply our newfound wellness education to our actual living! To echo the epigraph above, even though we cannot "count" wellness, our understanding of it can help us prioritize what counts in our life. This unfolds in several steps.

Begin by becoming the CEO (Chief Executive Officer) of your life. Even if business isn't your language, being the CEO of your being is an empowering concept to grasp. When we view the term through the lens of business-speak, we see that a company runs on the decision-making of the CEO who has to implement big-time solutions based on the most accurate information possible. This requires great flexibility in response to the chaos of consumer demands, shifts in the market, and the company's responsibility to stakeholders. Are you ready to take charge of your big business of wellness? Your body, mind, and spirit run on the winning decisions you make for you, others, and community. Take ownership of your company! You are the boss, leader, and head of state—your very own commander in chief.

How many times have we heard this one: "If only I could find a way to apply the discipline I have with _____ [fill in the blank] and apply it to exercise and diet!" How many successful executives do you know who are tigers in the boardroom but are chronically unhealthy and out of shape? Or what about the mother of three whose daily strategizing skills would put a three-star general to shame, but who never takes time to take care of herself?

In the next chapter, we'll meet "Client Two," who connected with her inner CEO and defined her health using parallel financial terms like temperance, discipline, and moderation. Client Two translated those words into targeted wellness terms she could sink her teeth into. In the wellness business, making lifestyle enhancements is about growth, not deficit.

Just as a CEO of a company cannot put minimal effort into running a business and expect success, you cannot expect to be well with insufficient sleep, a stressful work day without refreshment, and a dysfunctional personal life left unattended. You need a plan for success. A strategic plan prioritizes your values, vision, and mission. We are about to show you how to set doable goals and quickly analyze your strengths that will help you hit the bullseye.

What if business is not your language? Then use terms you can relate to. An artist might paint a visionary picture about what is important to life. An academic might turn to research, qualifying and quantifying a plan. An athlete might use parallel competition to increase his or her wellness: hard work, teamwork, tenacity, and never giving up. A musician might apply resonance and harmony into a well-being plan. The point is, we are each unique and can access the very best parts of ourselves to grow successfully in wellness. Happiness is not in our future, it's in our now. And strategizing wellness goals for ourselves is a great step in the right direction.

As we consider the process of setting goals, we have another helpful acronym for you. Goals need to be **SMART**: **S**pecific, **M**easureable, **A**chievable, **R**elevant, and **T**ime-based.

First, goals must be specific. Specific objectives have a much greater chance of being accomplished than general ones. Begin by stating your purpose and hoped-for benefits. For example, a general goal would be,

"Get in shape." But a specific goal would be, "Join the You Can Do It Fitness Club to improve stability, movement, and balance so I can enjoy my family"

Then, make your goals measurable so they can be quantified. An example might be, "I want to lose ten pounds," rather than "I want to lose weight."

An achievable goal is realistic to accomplish. For instance, it would probably not be realistic to say, "I will never eat sugar again." A more achievable goal might be "I will enjoy a moderate serving of sugar twice a week."

Is your goal relevant? Does it fit in with your Being Image mission? If, for example, your mission includes encouraging women to embrace their many beautiful body types, then "I want to look like a supermodel" won't fit.

Time-based goals have a beginning and an ending. Do you have a target date for completion? Calendar that particular date!

To make your goals even **SMARTER**, consider **E**motional **R**eadiness. Emotional readiness means you are empowered to start change. If any part of your plan is daunting, examine the blind spots, barriers, and burdens that may be making you feel this way. Does your plan have built-in breaks and recovery time so you can make improvements? If not, add them in. Does any part of your plan require additional strategies? If so, rewrite those parts. Is any part of your plan overly dependent on others? Revise it so you're the CEO in charge.

To give you some idea of how this can all play out, here are Andrew's SMART goals:

Family Goal	Build strong faith and trust in my family unit.
Faith Goal	Ground all my thoughts, words, and actions through wellness (an approach to communications we'll tell you more about in Chapter 7).
Happiness Goal	Utilize the foundation of my Being Image to illuminate others.

Health Goal	Honor my Being Image by experiencing movement throughout the fitness continuum and the four components of fitness.

What are your health and wellness goals? Better yet, what are your Being Image goals? Event goals are occasions like a 5K run, a basketball game, or bicycle race—or it may be the target date for reaching a physical fitness goal such as achieving 20% body fat, for example.

Strategies are the tactics that support adherence. Some examples are: attending aerobics class three times a week, engaging in a daily run, or adding power foods into the family diet. They are the "how to" processes that ensure smart goals are reached. Here are Andrew's daily strategies:

Family Strategies	Connect daily with my family by communicating from the very best part of myself; Inquire about their hopes and dreams for both self and others; Listen empathically to their feelings and opinions
Faith Strategies	Center my beingness through introspection; Create wellness energy by eating nourishing food; Illuminate others through ethical interactions
Happiness Strategies	Create a wellness perspective to my problems and their solutions; Reduce stress in problem situations by seeking dignified solutions; Reframe seemingly bad situations through meditation
Health Strategies	Perform 150 minutes of light to moderate physical activity per week; Alternate my favorite sports activities such as tennis, basketball, and jogging; Embrace activities of daily living through domestic and professional servitude; Prepare home cooked meals to promote family conversation five nights a week

Whatever your ambition, the important goals you define will guide your actions.

Remember the quote by John E. Lewis, "If not us, then who? If not now, then when?" We highly recommend writing strategies down as routine efforts. Andrew's goals and strategies are consistent with his life values. The goals are clearly defined, quantified, within reach, support the mission, and specified as daily. His strategies are defined to increase the likelihood of success. Yes, his goals and strategies are smart. And yours can be, too!

Now it's time to fill out the worksheet entitled "My SMART Goals" located in the Wellness in Mind Activities section.

Next, to maximize the effectiveness and efficiency of your plan, it can be very helpful to perform what is called a **SWOT analysis**. When we take a good look at our **S**trengths and **W**eaknesses, as well as the **O**pportunities and **T**hreats that face us, we have a much clearer vision of what we can accomplish, as well as a heads-up for the places we may fall down. One of the most helpful maxims to live by is "know yourself". A SWOT analysis encourages us to do just that. Forewarned is forearmed!

In preparation for a SWOT analysis, begin by creating a Life Line, which lists major events from first memories up and until present day. Revisiting significant life events allows people to identify past challenges and successes.

The next step is to list Life Guards, the most important and most influential people in your life. You may find the Life Guards in your life correspond quite closely with the experiences in your Life Line. Life events are often interspersed with remarkable people who served as safety nets of support, instilled in you valuable character traits, and aided your efforts to succeed.

Let's read Andrew's SWOT analysis first to get some helpful perspective. Using his Life Line and Life Guards, Andrew identifies his **S**trengths, **W**eakness, **O**pportunities and **T**hreats:

Strengths

Toughness and the ability to delay gratification within the systems of college football and higher education

Compassion, temperance, and empathy during conflict
(see Chapter 7's Gas Station Attendant Story)

Resilience, appreciation, and gratitude sustained my journey
back to health after my motorcycle accident

Being Image enhancement through the imitation of role models
Helen Garde, Dora Gomez, Mike Sheppard, and Dr.
Leon Griffin

Servitude within my roles as husband, father, government
employee, elected official, and philanthropist

Weaknesses

Winner-loser attachment patterns and familial distortions
developed during my upbringing

Opportunities

A positive Being Image to experience the human spirit in others
and illuminate the strengths of loved ones

Threats

Vexatious emotions and any social or physical environment that
diminishes my beingness and the beingness of others

Now is a good time to assess your challenges and find your go-to characteristics by completing "My SWOT Analysis" located in the Wellness in Mind Activities section.

Once you have your SWOT worksheet in hand, you can analyze it more closely to better define your strengths, weaknesses, opportunities, and threats. In the next chapter, we will show you how to respond to situations that trigger unhealthy behavior in your life. You will be empowered to reach for resilience!

The wonderful truth is that, if you are reading this book, you have experienced enough positive relating to establish a blueprint for wellness within your being. You can trust that blueprint for wellness to direct you toward what you are meant to be. It can provide purpose to living well, both within your being and through others. As we showed in Chapter 1, we are biologically imitating people. We're hard-wired to do it. In fact, we cannot *not* imitate. So the example we set for the world—our Being Image—is powerful. In fact, our Being Image cannot be resisted. We affect those around us simply by being. If you want, take another look at "Mirror Neurons" in the Appendix.

Remember the Socio-Ecological Model we showed you in Chapter 1? Ideally, we want to integrate all of our specific health and wellness actions within that Big Picture model since our wellness involves everyone in our world. Our context counts because we live not only within ourselves but also through others. We use the word *through* deliberately because neuroscience substantiates that we live through each other, changing each other as we do so, learning and coming into our beingness through intersubjective relating to each other. Our being is being-in-communion. Need a refresher on this? You may want to take another peek at "How We Are I-Other: Intersubjectivity" in the Appendix.

Pause to look at each level of the Socio-Ecological Model in "My Big Picture Worksheet" in the Wellness in Mind Activities section and ask yourself expansive questions for each one.

In excess, almost any action (or inaction) can diminish beingness, such as: eating unalive foods, negative emotions related to exercise, and social environments that diminish the spirit. When we move, fuel, and recharge we feel great. We also become strong enough to discard parts of our wellness business that are not performing as well as they should. Take a few minutes to reread all of your completed worksheets. Together, they are the tactical plan for your life-long business of wellness, your well-being plan for life. It's important to remember your well-being plan is dynamic; it changes as you change and as your life changes, so revisit it often, rethinking and rewriting it whenever you need to.

Envisioning your Being Image establishes a big picture. Developing SMART goals and weighing them against strengths, weaknesses, opportunities, and threats promotes your ability to target well-being for life. Taking a nonjudgmental look at your life events can uncover interesting facts about why you habitually do what you do. This discovery facilitates your moving through the early Processes of Change stage transitions described in the previous chapter.

Now it's time to learn how to reach for resilience when triggers tempt us. When we keep the Big Picture and our relationships in mind, we can truly begin to serve wellness to others.

Chapter 6

REACH for Resilience!

> Good timber doesn't grow with ease. The stronger the
> wind, the stronger the trees.
>
> —Douglas Malloch

Good results are what we seek by keeping wellness in mind. One way to grow positive results is resilience. We all experience stress at one time or another. Resilience is the ability to recover from it.

Physician Gabor Mate says, "Stress is a physiological response mounted by an organism when it is confronted with excessive demands on its coping mechanisms, whether biological or psychological. It is an attempt to maintain internal biological and chemical stability, or homeostasis, in the face of these excessive demands. The physiological stress response involves nervous discharges throughout the body and the release of a cascade of hormones, chiefly adrenaline and cortisol. Virtually every organ is affected, including the heart and lungs, the muscles, and, of course, the emotional centers in the brain. Cortisol itself acts on the tissues of almost every part of the body—from the brain to the immune system, from the bones to the intestines. It is an important part of the infinitely intricate system of checks and balances that enables the body to respond to the threat."[1]

Stress and our beliefs about it are correlated with illness.[2] To realistically perceive how much stress is in our life, the Holmes and Rahe Stress Scale contains a list of 41 events with values applied to each event according to stress level. We simply multiply the value by the number of times we have experienced each event in the last year to calculate our total stress level. Holmes and Rahe have found that a score of 150 gives us a 50-50 chance of developing an illness. You may want to take time to Google the Holmes and Rahe Stress Scale online and rate your stress level.

Stress is not bad in and of itself, but stress and our beliefs about it do affect us psychologically and biologically. And stress can affect relationships. Caregivers who are experiencing a stressful episode are prone to be less sensitive, more irritable, more critical, and more punitive with their children. Instead of modulating stimulation of their infants, they may induce very high levels of arousal in abuse and very low levels of arousal in neglect. If they provide no interactive repair, the infant's intense negative emotional states—states of emotional dissonance—last for long periods of time and can affect the infant's health.

The Adverse Childhood Experiences (ACE) Study[3] is a major American research project that poses the question of whether, and how, childhood experiences affect adult health decades later. The study makes it clear that time does not heal some of the adverse experiences of childhood. One does not "just get over" some things, even fifty years later.

The ACE study concentrates on three categories of childhood abuse and five categories of household dysfunction.

The three categories of abuse are:

> Recurrent physical abuse
> Recurrent severe emotional abuse
> Contact sexual abuse

The five household dysfunction categories are:

> Growing up in a household where someone was in prison
> Growing up in a household where the mother was treated violently
> Growing up with an alcoholic or drug user

> Growing up in a home where someone was chronically depressed, mentally ill, or suicidal
>
> Growing up in a home where at least one biological parent was lost to the patient during childhood – regardless of cause

The most important finding from the study is that adverse childhood experiences are more common than recognized or acknowledged and can have a powerful affect on adult health a half-century later.[4]

A distinction between abuse and dissonance is in order here. Abuse is never warranted; emotional dissonance is. Dissonance is important for socializing children. The parental "no" so common with two-year-olds is a valuable tool for protecting toddlers from harm. When the dissonance of the "no" is repaired—by showing the child he or she is loved despite the "no"—the experience stimulates the child's growth. It encourages a capacity for learning from and repairing the unavoidable dissonant experiences that we all encounter in life. It becomes a valuable tool that tells us when we are out of sync with ourselves or with another. Reparation of dissonance within resonance becomes the brain template for knowing how we can get ourselves back into harmony—the brain template for knowing how to regulate ourselves.

As brain scientist Donald Pfaff puts it, "The effects of stress hormones on behavior are not simple; they depend on whether or not the levels of those hormones have been elevated chronically and repeatedly. If not, that is, if stress has been rare, their effect is restorative: it brings the body's systems from an emergency state back toward a normal state. However—and this point is crucial—if the animal or human has been subjected to chronic fear and stress, the adrenal hormones summoned up again and again, then the steroidal stress hormones can destroy neurons and impede signaling pathways."[5]

So the question is: How can we build resilience to modulate and constructively harness our response to stress, which enhances our wellness?

We can reach for resilience with a helpful mechanism. Resilience is **R**ehearsed, **E**mpowered, **A**ctionable, **C**ollaborative, and **H**olistic. The acronym REACH helps us toward resilience by showing us how to overcome unhealthy behaviors without resorting to self-violence. In other words, we are not correcting a deficit, we are learning a new way of being. Thinking in deficit terms puts us into a tense state that doesn't help learning. Rather we want to learn new ways of being and in the process develop and reorganize our nervous systems and our brain.[6] A new way of being leads to a new way of behaving. Respect the natural ebb and flow of life and view its challenges, not as setbacks, but as learning experiences to hone your resilience skills. Instead of focusing on "good" or "bad" outcomes, just focus on your Being Image. Your actions will lead towards everything you desire.

REACH coincides seamlessly with the behavioral processes of change. The behavioral processes of change involve the activities people use to move into the action and maintenance stages of change (see "Later Stage Transitions—Processes of Change" described in Chapter 4). If you want to enhance your behaviors for wellness, REACH is the tool to do it.

Rehearsed Stimulus Control: Plan and prepare rehearsed responses to triggers that lead to problem behaviors. Visualize and practice strategies to ward off temptations within interpersonal, organizational, and community relationships.

When you're stuck at the family BBQ, fortify filler by adding tomato, spinach and onion to a burger. Enrich empty calories to ensure portion control. Eat an apple, for example, as a satiating snack before diving into the birthday cake. Keep satisfying live food within arm's reach at all times!

Empowered Counter Conditioning: Match the knowledge, skills, attitudes, and beliefs that have proven successful in the past to current wellness priorities. Empowered decisions derive from life values and an internal template for success, which grows with new knowledge and skills, with new attitudes and beliefs.

When temptation arrives, keep your life values at the forefront of decision-making. Learn from the role models around you that are consistent with your values. Take a firm stance on your desire for well-being by using devotionals, manifestos and mantras to steer wellness efforts.

Actionable Reinforcement Management: Calculate the potential gains and losses connected to problem behaviors. Target wellness actions based on a collaborative and holistic approach. Actionable means that decisions do not remain a mere thought, wish, or empty promise. When temptation looms, life values rule and our expression of wellness is clear to self and others through determined action.

When triggered, asked the following questions: How did previous decisions play out with regard to the six dimensions of wellness? What were the gains and losses? Is there a high risk for a fleeting reward in your current situation? Ground yourself in wellness by assessing where you are, what time it is, what you want, what responsibilities require you to be your best the next day and, most importantly, who depends on your wellness in order to be well themselves.

Collaborative Helping Relationships: Resilience is inclusive of the family, faith, happiness, and health continuum. Disclose the actions you want to enhance to trusted advocates. Keep the successes from your Life Line in mind and always have your Life Guards on speed dial.

Call a friend who enjoys basketball and set up a game. Reach out to families and plan a potluck dinner. Schedule a weekly gardening day with neighbors to cultivate natural produce.

Holistic Beingness Liberation: A holistic conviction enhances our beingness and the beingness of others through the six Big Picture Dimensions of Wellness (physical, occupational, social, intellectual, emotional, and spiritual). This commitment strengthens the rehearsed, empowered, actionable, and collaborative responses that lead to resilience. Engage in the small but meaningful task of acknowledging others with gratitude. This gains trust and earns respect. When you experience someone acting like a bad apple, do not get spoiled in his or her neurology; connect with his or her goodness and create new beingness.

Reaching for resilience calls us to face our fears. In facing fears we can change our being from living in a body-state of fear to living in a body-state of calm. In so doing we can change our behavior from maladaptive to healthy.

THE BIOLOGY OF FEAR-BASED BEHAVIOR

Brain scientist Donald Pfaff describes the process of fear-based behavior this way: Experiencing fear begins with sensory signals. Signals of smell and sight reach the amygdala directly. The other senses go up the brain stem to the thalamus. From the thalamus, some signals go to the amygdala; others go first to the cerebral cortex and then to the amygdala. Thereafter the message "be afraid" is distributed to other brain regions in order to coordinate our responses to it. The message to the hippocampus affects our memory of fear; the message to the hypothalamus elicits our urge to fight; the message to the area of the brain called locus coeruleus elicits the feeling of fear; and the message to the midbrain central grey results in sweating, shallow breathing and rapid heart rate. "Thus, signals from the amygdala produce the emotional body language of fear, and this language appears to reflect each person's individual temperament or character."[7]

At times, fear can be lifesaving: think of our human flight response to encountering a seedy character with a knife, for example. But when fear arises from dread laid down in brain templates of unrepaired dissonant or traumatic experiences, fear can be difficult to deal with. Such fear may take different forms:

> We may fear losing the person who threatens us.
> We may fear losing that person's love or approval.
> We may fear punishment by that person.
> We may establish unrealistic ideals and fear not living
> up to them.

Whatever the form of our fear, we develop fear-based behaviors in our attempt to cope with threatening others whom we nonetheless need. Fear affects our function in predictable ways:[8]

> Non-traumatic unrepaired dissonance—such as being
> misunderstood—puts us in a subjective state of arousal
> or alarm (fight/flight). In this fight/flight body-state, our
> cognitive style becomes concrete. Our emotional brain
> regulates us; we have no access to our higher neocortical
> cognitive functions.

Traumatic dissonance—such as physical or sexual abuse—puts us in a subjective state of terror. In this body-state our cognitive style is reflexive and our brain stem (automatic) level regulates us.

Stated differently, "People process, store and retrieve information and then respond to the world in a manner that depends upon their current physiological state (in other words, their response is 'state-dependent')....a calm child [person] will process information very differently from one who is in an 'alarmed' state . . . Even if two children [people] have identical IQs, the calmer child [person] can more readily focus on the words of the teacher and, using her neocortex, engage in abstract thought and learning. In contrast, the child [person] who is alarmed will be less efficient at processing and storing the verbal information the teacher is providing."[9]

Fear-based behaviors become problematic when we use them excessively and lock ourselves into rigid reactions of maladaptive behaviors. The good news is that we can change our biology from fear to calm.

Here are Seven Steps for Facing Fears and Building Resilience[10]

1. **Awakening**: Becoming aware of how our fear-based behavior results in maladaptive ways of connecting with others physically, psychologically, and spiritually. Very simply this means waking up to our blind spots, barriers, and burdens.

2. **Naming**: Articulating our fear-based behavior within a mutually interactive relationship of trust. Naming invites us to see how our fear-based behavior once had survival value because it organized our understanding, diminished our pain, and kept us in relationship. Naming also invites us to see how this behavior now limits us, diminishing our resilience. Because we come into being through another, we bring our fear-based behavior into relationship with a trusted other in order to change our being.

3. **Accepting**: Accepting acknowledgment of our fear-based behavior by the trusted other. We need someone to acknowledge our naming. Accepting their acknowledgment moves us to the side of our trusted other so that we can address the fear-based behavior together.

4. **Repenting**: Allowing ourselves to be sorry for our fear-based behavior and allowing our minds to be changed. Allowing ourselves to feel sorry does not mean blaming our self. It is realizing that when we live in fear, we diminish our self and others. We diminish our wellness.

5. **Forgiving**: Forgiving the person with whom we established the fear-based behavior and living into the forgiveness of ourselves for the consequences of our behavior. Reaching resilience may or may not involve forgiveness by the person with whom we developed the fear-based behavior. It may be a third person—therapist, fitness trainer, or friend—who pronounces forgiveness. But reaching resilience must ultimately involve our forgiveness *of* that person. It must also involve our living into the forgiveness of our self that has been given by another. Through the eyes of the other we come into our being.

6. **Choosing well-being**: Choosing well-being moves us to an acceptance of the fact that our fear-based behavior came from mutual brokenness. Now the forgiving person can intentionally journey from fear back to resilience.

7. **Embracing, and being embraced by, goodness**: The sensation of embracing our natural goodness is what we feel when we become free from the bondage of fear. It is being good. In wellness terms, being good signals resilience. Having achieved resilience, we can now use our goodness to serve wellness to others.

But first, let us see how Andrew's Client Two achieved resilience.

Client Two

When she was fifteen, Client Two survived a horrific accident and was told she would probably never walk again. While she did walk again, she underwent many surgeries on her right leg, including a knee replacement when she was in her forties. Now, a widow in her late-sixties, she sought me out to focus on wellness and find new meaning in her life. Together we developed a well-being plan.

As part of the well-being plan, I sent her for stability and mobility work at the Institute of Community Wellness and Athletics (ICWA). After four months, she gained three pounds of muscle and lost four pounds of fat. The staff at ICWA were elated and Client Two was reveling in her results: she could walk up stairs without pain and she could now lift herself out of a chair without steadying herself with her upper body. She enjoyed movement in a way she hadn't in years.

Client Two created age-appropriate goals of physical stability and mobility and through the introspective work of Wellness in Mind she recreated her Being Image.

She declared her current purpose and chronicled her Life Line. She reflected on glorious victories and trials and tribulations. She wrote about her Life Guards, listing people who played a substantial part in her beingness. Lastly, she detailed the "how" of her well-being plan by balancing stability and mobility SMART goals with a SWOT analysis. The result was a practical and realistic plan with strategies to employ in times of weakness. In order to reframe turbulent emotional experiences, Client Two also planned and practiced situational confidence. In the end she was able to predict where she might be tempted and to focus her mind on envisioning how she would respond with confidence. She could reach for resilience whenever she recognized it was needed. The total well-being process and subsequent journaling revealed her great strengths. She came up with many positive and motivating declarations. While some of them are specific to her, others are so inspiring that you may want to incorporate them into your own well-being plan. Here is Client Two's plan:

My mission is to be as healthy and productive as possible. People are like oxygen to me. I am mentally strong.

Life Line

My bumps in the road have strengthened me. I was told I would never walk again, but I still had a leg and did not know why I could not walk on it. In times of heartbreak, a psychiatrist's couch was the best money I ever spent. I've bought two homes that hold cherished memories for me.

I married a dear man and became a stepmother to a great young lady; she is my sister-daughter.

Mom, without a doubt, is the strongest person I have ever known; she was the glue that kept our family together. In the year 2000, I recovered well from four surgeries. Rejection stinks but I cannot and will not force friendship. I like to take trips, drink a cup of coffee, watch a few favorite TV shows, sit and hold hands, and sometimes savor a bit of ice cream. I can bowl, swim, and twirl a baton. I have experienced great jobs and careers; I have been the CEO of a company.

Life Guards

After listing the champions in her life she wrote: "Those are the ones who are near and dear to my heart—the very people I will depend on and reflect with to deepen my purpose of being as healthy and productive as possible. Attributes I admire and model are: integrity, patience, self-motivation, dependability, strength, resourcefulness, positivity, and loyalty. I admire being real, responsible, intelligent, independent, confident, and honest. I am chief executive officer of me."

We have already discussed how empowering it is to adopt the title of CEO for our own life. When she really experienced this, Client Two claimed her rightful place as the person in charge of her well-being.

PART III

INTERSUBJECTIVITY: PLAY WELL WITH OTHERS TO CO-CREATE LIFE AND HEALTH

This last section explores ways to cultivate wellness in all aspects of personal and professional life. By stimulating your own unique means to co-create with and through others, you'll truly have Wellness in Mind.

Chapter 7

Serving Wellness to Others

> Everything that irritates us about others can lead us to an understanding of ourselves.
>
> —Carl Jung

In reaching for resilience, we have essentially lived the truth of Swiss psychoanalyst Carl Jung's insight, looking at irritations derived from childhood conditioning as opportunities to co-create a new Being Image of our body, mind, and spirit. And when we do that, we know that new Being Image is a means to provide goodness through each other. In other words, we have nourished our life so that we can give it away.

There are two directions that wellness expansion can go, and our being knows them both: vertical (righting our self) and horizontal (righting others). Having righted our self, we can now serve wellness to our community by welcoming opportunities to connect with others and help them right their selves.

Giving truly is the secret of living!

To use another corporate parallel, business success depends on business-to-business and business-to-client relationships. A large retail chain includes many affiliations with sourcing, shipping, warehousing, distribution, retailing, and end-consumer marketing. Any break in this value-chain of productivity can result in failure.

The business of being is similar. As physically well as we can make our own body, we are still dependent on others for positive energy flow. The people around us, the places we are in, and the foundation on which we interact greatly affect our wellness value chain: the quality of the goodness we share with others.

Let's begin serving wellness to others by recalling **POSIES**, the National Wellness Institute's Six Dimensions of Wellness: **P**hysical, **O**ccupational, **S**ocial, **I**ntellectual, **E**motional and **S**piritual. Within each of the six dimensions of wellness, here is what expanding wellness looks like:[1]

Physical: The benefits of regular physical activity, healthy eating habits, strength and vitality as well as personal responsibility, self-care, and knowing when to seek medical attention constitute the absolute linchpin for success in wellness existence. A plan for physical wellness, for example, readies us to be the human mirror for others to come into their own being.

Occupational: The enrichment of life through work and its interconnectedness to living and playing touches self and others.

Social: A person contributes to their environment and community and builds better living spaces and social networks. Contributions to environment, community, and better living spaces are inclusive of social networks.

Intellectual: Creative and stimulating mental activities and sharing our gifts uplifts others.

Emotional: Self-esteem, self-control, and determination give a sense of direction. This sense of purpose is dependent upon the familial relationships and friendships formed since the day we were born.

Spiritual: The development of belief systems, values, and creating a world-view denotes how we learn through others to co-create win-win exchanges where benevolence prevails for all.

Each wellness dimension involves interrelatedness—relating or connecting through another—as a practice within the realm. People are attracted to growth and by helping others be better we become an attraction of goodness. Attraction is the portal through which we arrive at opportunities for positive personal interactions with others.

There is an old Russian tale about the inhabitants of heaven and hell. The inhabitants in both places sit at tables loaded with delicious food, but they can only eat with extremely long-handled forks that they must grasp at the end of the handle. The inhabitants of hell starve because they cannot figure out how to feed themselves. The inhabitants in heaven thrive by reaching across the table and feeding each other, knowing the reciprocity of beingness. This story is a kind of template: with wellness in mind, we too can engage in non-rivalrous, mutually influencing, co-creating processes that nourish ourselves and others.

Our attitudes and beliefs, together with our knowledge and skills, can assist us in serving wellness to others. In doing so, the manner in which we communicate is vitally important for creating empathic relationships at home, work, and community. Here are a few questions to help you clarify your interactions with others:

> What is my internal motivation in discourse?
> What intentions derive from my motivations?
> What circumstances in my personal and professional life
> affect my motivations and intentions?
> What is my final expectation?

At the forefront of social motivation is a wish to belong. Theologian James Alison writes, "Someone *belongs* whose sense of being is peacefully dependent on the regards of those with whom they live."[2] Such a sense of being can only exist where people are being creatively *for* each other without being *against* each other in any way.

We communicate with intentions of what we are trying to accomplish through our interactions. Intentions that are non-rivalrous come from *being* good—of self-giving gratuitously to others and receiving compassionately from others. Collaborative expectations focus on win-win results for all persons involved.

We can only realize true collaboration if we pay attention to what is actual, real, and true for the other. Here are three simple steps for win-win communication:

Acknowledge and Ask: Reach out to others by introducing yourself and inquiring about their life. Attune to their answers with an open and empathic heart. Fight the temptation to dive into your wants and needs (or thoughts

71

about what the other person should do). By inviting others into your own positive neurology you share common happiness on dignified ground.

Inform and Involve: Empower others with factual information and, if at all possible, back it up with data. Avoid blaming, excuses, and empty promises. Invite others who share your interests to engage. An influential person with a willing spirit attracts opportunities for co-creation.

Clarify and Connect: Ensure solid understanding by paraphrasing and summarizing messages. Take action to identify a "next step" and calendar the follow up. Express gratitude for the opportunity to collaborate with the people involved.

Wellness change is about positivity. Life becomes easier as we develop a dignified way of interacting with others, but we have to accept that conflict between people is par for the course and that, in moments of unrest, emotional reactions often outrank social mores. When conflicting intentions exist, learning how to de-escalate conflict can be helpful. Remember, with every conflict there is opportunity to reestablish our Being Image of why we are here in the world.

VERBAL DEFENSE AND INFLUENCE

Verbal Defense and Influence training is the skill of verbally redirecting negative behavior with presence and words.[3] Persuasion is based on several premises.

Response versus Reaction: If someone behaves angrily towards us and we become angry in return, we are simply mirroring; we are becoming like them and perpetuating negative behavior. If, however, we keep our self in a body-state of calm, we can respond out of selfless concern for the well-being of the other. This can de-escalate anger and redirect negative behavior.

Ethical Presence: We can meet unexpected indignities that characterize aggressive human interactions by establishing a calm mindset through a strong body posture and deep breathing. A calm mindset can enable us to *be* creatively *for* the others rather than *against* them.

Voice: Match voice with ethical presence. A focus on peaceful resolve must be heard through our pitch, pace, tone, facial expressions and body movements. Being Image is maximized as the voice seamlessly matches the message.

These communication skills set the stage for verbal defense and influence. Our efforts to serve wellness to others can be helped by using five steps of persuasion to generate compliance, cooperation, and collaboration from people in crisis.

The trainers at the Vistelar Group, a global speaking and training organization focused on addressing human conflict, have worked on persuasion skills since the early 1980s. Their primary purpose is to keep people safe by teaching them how to prevent conflict from occurring, how to verbally de-escalate conflict if it does occur, and how to defend themselves physically if they are attacked. As with all best-laid plans, circumstances trump disposition and when conflict arises it's best to persuade people to do the right thing, especially when they are resistant. The following steps provide a compelling argument to convince others to make good decisions.

Uphold Dignity – Show Respect: Dignity is recognition of the life value of self and all others as an objective, intrinsic, and inalienable right. Respect avoids harm or interference with that right by showing an unconditional positive regard for self and others. Respect begins with an ethical presence of valuing others and others see it the second we walk in the door.

Make a Request – Avoid Barking Orders: A request invites a response. Barking orders signals disrespect and diminishment of the other. Tactical communications experts know that almost all people would rather be asked rather than told to do something. A professional greeting precedes the ask, "Hello, my name is Gary and I am in charge of the sales floor. I noticed you are on a personal phone; would you please place it in your locker until your shift is over?"

Declare the Context – Based on Rules: To declare context is to announce the circumstances that explain why a person should behave a certain way. The rules of the organization protect both the employee and the leader. For example, "Our mission to provide excellent customer service doesn't support phone use" (Note: if the rules aren't being followed by the majority, the organization should revisit them).

Give Options – Avoid Threats: Giving options helps a person make the best choice for their self. Sometimes this means pointing out a bad choice. For example, "You can choose to put the phone away or select disciplinary action. Your work has been improving and you are valued. I don't want disciplinary action for you; do you really need this added burden?"

Offer a Second Chance: Address non-compliant behavior as an advocate. This includes respectfully discussing strategies to turn things around. For example, "I know you're upset about the inefficiencies of the group, but expressing it as non-compliant phone use will lead to discipline. Let's work together to formalize your complaint in a productive manner."

The surprising secret of the five steps for persuasion is that, by remaining in the role of advocate, we can literally draw others into our neurology of influence. A closer look at the steps of persuasion demonstrates how others imitate us not only physically, but also by their adopting our character values and strengths:

When you uphold the dignity of the other, the other imitates you. A secure attachment bond is initiated.

A request delivered in a respectful voice establishes rapport. The person can begin to see, hear, and feel understood. The person is invited to believe in you.

Explaining policy transmits clarity and assists in decision-making. By declaring the context of a request, the other is invited to believe in the system.

When an advocate presents options as an opportunity to do the right thing, the seeds of critical thinking are planted. The person begins to believe in him or her self.

By offering a second chance, consideration is shown for the suffering and misfortune of the other. By treating the other as an equal, the person feels equal and believes in compassion.

The results are valuable: as persuasion steps are consistently delivered, the neurology of influence builds positive beliefs and better attitudes in others.

While these steps are commonly taught in compliance-driven industries with black-and-white institutional imperatives (such as public safety, criminal justice, and healthcare), they can pave the way for ethical interaction in all parts of life. The elderly and the young especially need our cooperation and collaboration.

Here's some wellness food for thought: Through ethical interaction and influence we can begin to enrich, fortify, and refine relationships with the young and the mature. Make the world of the elderly a better place and they, with their wisdom, can help us put our worries in proper perspective. Children need tons of love and encouragement to grow their Being Images. We can deliver fair counsel and advocacy to help them become peaceful adults. In return, they can bring us acceptance.

Andrew's Gas Station Attendant Story is a short tale of how he overcame conflict and anger to serve wellness to someone else.

Gas Station Attendant Story

The incident begins at quarter past seven in the morning of September 25, 2003—five years to the day before the motorcycle accident that changed my life forever. I am all pumped up from a weight lifting session at the Westside Community Center. I leave the gym and jump into my white Ford Ranger. I get halfway home before looking down at the gas gauge.

Damn. I could easily have stopped by the Diamond Shamrock and filled up last night. What shall I do? My truck is running on fumes!

My money is on my dresser at home. I park in front of my house, run in, grab the cash and run back out. Roman's Gas Station is just around the corner. I pull up and it's closed, but the sign on the door reads "Open 7:30 am." The clock in my truck says 7:26 am. *I won't make it to another station,* I think to myself. *Oh, well, the station is almost open.*

I buy a newspaper. Many minutes pass as I read about Arnold Schwarzenegger's first political debate and ESPN's new fishing show starring Deion Sanders. When I glance up, I see the Coca Cola deliveryman stacking product next to the locked-up gas station door.

Finally, the gas station attendant arrives. By now, I'm talking to myself. *Boy, do I want to give her a piece of my mind! I'm going to be late for work because of her!*

My truck door is open. I hear this tardy lady tell the deliveryman that she first needs to count her money, so I sit for another few minutes in my truck. As I walk into the station, she looks at me and blurts out:

"You're going to have to wait awhile. I still have to open my drawer."

I respond with a matter of fact, "I've been waiting for fifteen minutes."

She glares at me. "I don't care if you've been waiting."

I grit my teeth and feign calm, "You don't care? You should care. I'm a customer."

"I said I don't care."

"You should care. I'm the customer and I've been waiting for . . ."

She interrupts, "I don't care if you've been waiting for half an hour. I've had a very bad morning and if you keep giving me a hard time, I don't have to serve you."

I try to keep my cool, "I'm not giving you a hard time. I'm stating a fact—I've been waiting here for fifteen minutes."

"You can go somewhere else!"

"I can't go anywhere else! I'm out of gas!"

I am beside myself with anger, pumped up with caffeine and adrenaline from coffee and weight lifting. Ugly thoughts are running through my head. *Nasty! Tardy! Bitter! Rude! Low-life loser! I'll never set foot in here again!*

The attendant finally gets the cash drawer in order and gives me eye contact. I can't believe my next words as I hand her a ten-dollar bill...

"Ten on pump four, please."

The second I say it I regret it. I couldn't believe I said "please" after everything she put me through! My mind races: *Oh, man. Why did I put $10 in? I should have put $2 so I could spend the rest of my good money at another station. I'm going to write a nasty letter to the manager of this place. But with my luck, she's probably a relative of the person in charge—that's why she thinks she can act like that.*

As I drive home, I recall everything that has transpired. In the midst of my recollections, I remember that a few months earlier my supervisor, Joanne Caffrey, had loaned me a book on meditation. One of the emotions it addressed was anger. It advised that, when angry, put that anger in a pot and let it boil. Then respond instead of react. *I sure let it boil this morning,* I thought.

Then, something or someone within my Being Image suggested, "Say a prayer for her. Better yet, write her a note telling her that she was prayed for today."

Yes, that's it! I bet I can make this a win-win situation.

When I arrive home, I get on the computer and go to Microsoft Publisher:

New Document *CLICK*
Greeting Cards *CLICK*
Sympathy Cards *CLICK*
Best Wishes *CLICK*
Nice graphic, I thought. *DOUBLE-CLICK!* I start typing…

"You have been prayed for this morning. I hope the rest of your day goes well."

—Andrew

As I get dressed for work, I can't help but think: *This note may be just a little bit corny for my personality.* But as I leave home, I decide to go with it.

My appearance is much improved now that I'm in a suit and tie. Perhaps this might make a positive difference and I ponder my approach, *Will she recognize me? Do I say anything or just give her the note?* I answer myself with residual anger.

It probably doesn't matter what I do. She's so nasty she might just rip it up without reading it.

I enter the gas station and see her behind the counter. I smile. She immediately recognizes me and smiles back. For one split second it seems we are sharing the same ridiculous joke.

"I'm sorry," she offers.

"It's OK," I counter. "This is for you," and I hand her the folded note.

After she reads it, words tumble out of her mouth as she grasps her shoulder, "Thank you. I'm sorry but I might have a tumor in my shoulder and I have to go back to the doctor and I'm scared of what he's going to find."

Without forethought I put one hand on her shoulder. The other hand holds hers and I say, "It's okay. Everything will be alright because people are praying for you."

Her eyes well up with tears as she repeatedly thanks me and apologizes. When another customer walks in, the attendant wipes away her tears. Seeing that she is composed, I say, "take care" and leave.

What a beautiful human exchange! It was so moving I had to dab my eyes with tissue on the way to work. I found myself smiling at grumpy rush-hour drivers, allowing lane-changers to cut in front of me, arriving at work and greeting my employees without doling out an assignment or a lecture about policies and procedures. I was hearing and seeing my surroundings with a new clarity and a new mission: to make the most out of every human exchange.

It's easy to react and treat people as hatefully as they treat us. The challenge is to respond with compassion. To love when someone isn't being lovable. To change the hate inside one's heart into love and send that love to another.

I visit my friend again about a month later. The first words out of her mouth are, "Where have you been? I've been waiting and waiting for you. I think about you every day."

Giving her a hug, I ask how she is.

With a big smile on her face she says, "You're my guardian angel. My shoulder is healed."

I feel overjoyed. We chat briefly and give each other another wonderful hug goodbye. Our friendship continues to this day. I am forever her "Angel."

Chapter 8

Wellness in the World

> The key to growth is the introduction of higher dimensions
> of consciousness into our awareness.
>
> —Lao Tzu

As we come to the end of our wellness journey together we want to underscore a vitally important fact once again: we shape and are shaped by intersubjective connection. Our Being Image is never autonomous; we are never separate as we sometimes might wish we were. Instead, because we are beings who automatically and non-consciously imitate, we *are* what we imitate. We are I-Other beings. In other words, we are in relationship—in union—from our beginning, which produces our being. Depending on who we imitate, we can be compassionate or violent beings. So we must be mindful of what and who we imitate since, inevitably, that is what we will embody.

In the spirit of compassion and wellness for the world, our all-inclusive objective is to instill health within and throughout *all* environments. We can do this by using the key Lao Tzu mentions above: higher dimensions of consciousness. Psychologist Kenneth J. Gergen names that higher dimension of consciousness "relational consciousness."[1] As relational beings, he writes, "[W]e may abandon the view that those around us cause our actions. Others are not the causes or we their effects. Rather, in whatever we think, remember, create, and feel, we *participate* in relationship."[2]

In our modern society the social networks we participate in have grown ever larger and more discordant. Now our networks expand beyond family, friends and colleagues, into e-relationships through social media. Increasingly we are interrelated around our entire world, which has become more populated, more multicultural, and more mobile. Because we are more interrelated, it is more necessary than ever that we live cooperatively.

An example of approaching health through a global socio-ecological lens can be found in *The New Mexico Plan to Promote Healthier Weight*. This demonstration of inclusive relational consciousness can expand our vision of wellness, going beyond the individual to encompass the world.

The New Mexico Plan to reduce obesity, overweight, and related chronic diseases was created by a statewide collaborative of over 150 partners in New Mexico. The University of New Mexico Prevention Research Center and the New Mexico Department of Health Physical Activity & Nutrition Program coordinated the plan for Healthier Weight, with funding provided through a cooperative agreement with the Centers for Disease Control and Prevention, Division of Nutrition and Physical Activity.

This model of collaboration raises consciousness about health beyond individual lifestyles, showing how programs at the public policy, community, and organizational levels can support the interpersonal level. The plan sets forth objectives for changes to be made in six settings:[3]

Community and Regional Planning: "This setting includes coalitions, citizens, and community leaders as well as planners, developers and governments whose efforts focus on local policies related to physical infrastructure (such as roads, sidewalks, activity trails, parks, community gardens, as well as access to parks, grocery stores, and other businesses). Programs may include community-based activities, advocacy in support of funding for non-motorized transportation, or support of coalitions whose goals include improving the accessibility of healthful food or 'walkability' in communities."[4]

Within the overarching sphere of public policy, much community and regional planning is done at the federal, state, and local levels of government. Most Americans are involved in public policy through voting, yet are minimally drawn to policy at the grass-roots-action level. While individual callings may not lead us to become policy makers, engaged citizenry surely maximizes those efforts.

For some information about the philanthropic organization Rotary International as a paradigm of engaged citizenry, see "The Rotary Club: Andrew's Engaged Citizenry In Action" in the Appendix.

Education Systems: "This setting includes public and private schools for K-12, pre-kindergarten, day care and higher educational systems including technical and vocational schools, community colleges and universities. Interventions may focus on the students themselves (such as classes that are provided on physical activity and nutrition) or may address the various environments to support healthful nutrition and physical activity."[5]

Some predict that physical education at the federal, state, and local government levels will return from the current state of "stack them deep and teach them cheap" to become a rigorous requirement throughout all levels of education. Unit plans will, hopefully, include a health concepts approach with life skills based on wellness principles. The effort will build a larger school wellness culture that addresses teacher stress and enhances wellness throughout the school community.

INQUIRIES FOR TODAY'S PHYSICAL EDUCATION

Andrew has observed a social dynamic within physical education classes focused primarily on competitive team sports. According to his observation as a student teacher, the top 20% of students in traditional physical education classes seem to have an absolute blast. The next 30% of students, while they are not at the top of the class, are still performing at satisfactory levels and receive positive feedback about their abilities. That's the good news.

The sad reality is that one in every two students (the bottom 50%) in traditional physical education is not enjoying the experience. Instead they are being exposed to repetitive lose-lose situations. Any biological success through calories burned or homeostasis realized is being defeated by negative emotional feedback. The results are low self-esteem, low self-efficacy, and negative attitudes and beliefs about themselves and about movement and play in general. Hopefully, a holistic and collaborative approach to physical education suggested by the questions below can serve as an integrated wellness movement in our school systems. In order to introduce integrated physical wellness programs in public schools that meet the emotional needs of all students, school administrators must ask:

What are the psychological effects of physical education today?

What are the physical, social, and emotional experiences of the children?

How does their physical education experience relate to the six dimensions of wellness?

What are the internalized attitudes and beliefs about physical education in both staff and students?

How can teachers and administrators in the education setting adopt the facts of neuroscience as motivation to create collaborative role modeling?

How can we mirror contemporary advances in the fitness industry in order to expand the teaching parameters of physical education, health, and nutrition into a school-wide wellness culture?

Explore physical education excellence at: shapeamerica.org

Families and Communities: "This setting focuses on the support structures of family groups and individuals and peers within their respective communities. Healthy behaviors are created and facilitated when strategies include support by family members and peers. Interventions may target environmental factors as well as interpersonal and behavioral patterns affecting family and community members. Programs may include educational sessions on health, goal setting, problem-solving, family behavioral management, and community-wide initiatives."[6]

FAMILY AND COMMUNITY WELLNESS CONVERSATIONS

Within the family environment, we can create emotionally safe connections around the dinner table and through collaborative play. Invite children into conversations through open-ended inquiry. Drs. Bill Miller and Stephen Rollnick, the originators of Motivational Interviewing, use the acronym OARS to draw out answers from your children, family members, and friends:

Open-ended questions like, "What was lunch like for you today?"

Affirmations such as, "Feeding your body right is a main reason you feel so good!"

Reflective listening for example, "It sounds like you did yourself some good! Tell me more."

Summarizing as in, "You are honoring the food you are so privileged to have."

Families and communities do well to remain engaged in the wellness conversation. Such exchanges can unite the beingness health of your family with like-spirited community members through your local education system, community and regional planning efforts, and influential food systems. The following questions may be helpful as we seek to expand wellness efforts:

- How can I create a respectful family forum within which to share, laugh, and cry?
- How can I integrate the collective talents of my family into the larger community?

Learn about MI training at: motivationalinterviewing.org

Food Systems: "This setting includes the production, distribution, marketing and availability of foods and beverages. Interventions may target the availability and-or cost of healthful food choices in grocery stores, restaurants, vending machines, farmers markets, food banks, and food stamp or food voucher programs."[7]

INTERACTING AROUND FOOD

Theorists such as Noam Chomsky have argued that systematic bias exists in modern media.[8] Television, Internet, and social media provide more sensory-specific experience than printed ads. They target sight where everyone and everything looks perfect in unrealistic social occasions and sound, where laughter and music evoke feelings and orators describe irresistible tastes. As we presented in Chapter 3, the goal of advertising is to create allure through instant gratification of individual wants and of individual needs for love and belonging.

Social media takes marketing to another objectifying level by inviting people to participate in cyber-socialization. Burgers are not only looking bigger on TV, but customers can proudly post photos of their meal on social media. Participants become indoctrinated at every level of the socio-ecological model. As a nation, we become easily deceived. In our informational society, we need to re-introduce the essentials of human interaction, such as acknowledgement, gratitude, and compassion.

One way to do this is to select foods that are nourishing and flavorful using the 3SP acronym (Salt, Sugar, Saturated fat; Product, Preparation, Promotion) from Chapter 3. In this way, rather than mindlessly following the dictates of advertising, we are interacting thoughtfully with our food.

Navigate food systems at: cspinet.org

We've all been told to eat our fruits and veggies. As we mentioned in Chapter 3, delicious live food is not as easily marketed as food-like products, especially in the fast food industry. We can keep fighting the good fight with a couple of wonderful examples of wellness in action just as Andrew did when he found two tasty recipes by chance during his travels. They both blend (literally) super foods from the fruits and vegetables isle.

In 2011, I was on a plane to Milwaukee, Wisconsin and ended up sitting between an eighty-five year old gentleman named Mac and his wife Marlene. We spoke about careers, family, education and illness. Then Mac told me about a salsa he and his friend, Brock, created. They call it Mac-Brock Salsa and it sounded so good that I immediately made a batch when I returned to Albuquerque. I loved it and have dabbled with the ingredients ever since:

1 habanero chile
8 Roma tomatoes
1 medium red or white onion
1 bunch cilantro
3 cloves garlic
1 lime (juiced)
1 tsp. salt

Dice and mix ingredients together, cover with plastic wrap, place in the refrigerator and let marinate overnight.

By opening up my being to another, an otherwise insignificant encounter turned into a pleasant human connection and a shared recipe for a popular southwestern staple chock-full of power foods!

The second recipe is an almond butter smoothie from Outside magazine that I picked up in Salt Lake City (I grabbed it to read the cover story about an amputee athlete):

1 cup strawberries
1/2 cup milk
1/2 scoop (10 grams) undenatured whey protein
1/2 tablespoon coconut oil
1 tablespoon honey
1 tablespoon almond butter (or 2 tablespoons almonds)

Place all ingredients in a blender or food processor. Blend until smooth, then add ice and blend again until thick and frothy. This smoothie yields 370 calories, 42 grams of carbohydrate, and 14 grams of protein (as a matter of personal taste, I skip on the whey protein and substitute natural peanut butter).

We highly recommend exploring your community's food systems with curiosity. You can begin by asking:

How can I differentiate between food-like products and real live food?

Is most of the food in my favorite grocery store shipped in or
locally-grown and produced?

Farmers markets are becoming increasingly popular in urban
areas. Where are the ones nearest to me?

If you have a green thumb, help children plant foods like tomatoes,
cucumbers, and green beans. The reward is great, as they taste the work of
their own hands. They will grow in appreciation of the hard work it takes
to put food on the table and will also learn the importance of sharing fuel
and nourishment with others.

Healthcare Systems: "This setting may include health care providers,
staff and administrators, health care settings (offices, clinics, school-
based health centers, hospitals); training programs (university programs
in medicine, nursing, nutrition, behavioral health, exercise physiology);
health care systems and payors (managed care organizations, Medicare,
Medicaid, Veterans Administration, military, Indian Health Service, fee
for service plans); and purchasers of health insurance (employers and
individuals). Interventions may address affordability of and access to health
care services for patients, training and/or provision of resources to health
care providers, and health system changes that support promotion of
healthier weight in clinical settings."[9]

ASSESSING OUR RISK

The medical industry, much like the food industry, is ruled by revenue.
Revenue in the medical industry is earned by addressing health symptoms
because it is our behavior born of ignorance, denial or negligence that is
responsible for most diseases.

Technological advances seem to be both helping and hurting the
masses. The positive is that advances such as arthroscopic procedures have
minimized the trauma and risk of invasive surgeries of the past. However,
medical marvels such as joint replacements can be pushed on patients
before physical therapy is sought out, even though "physical therapy has
been shown to improve function and may delay or prevent the need for
knee replacement."[10]

When accessed correctly, there is more good than bad in healthcare systems. Consistent check-ups are helpful. An annual exam includes a review of family history to identify genetic predisposition for disease, a review of overall body functions including blood pressure and blood work, cholesterol levels and A1C test (reflects average blood sugar level for the past two to three months). An annual exam is also an opportunity to consult with a primary care physician about health risk behaviors and how to break them.

A health risk assessment (also called a health risk appraisal or well-being assessment) is a questionnaire based on behaviors proven to have a causal effect on health. An honest account of current behaviors such as smoking, caffeine intake, prescription and illicit drug use, alcohol consumption and amounts of salt, sugar, and saturated fat in the diet makes the appraisal a useful assessment tool for monitoring health. When assessing health risk, ask yourself:

> What behaviors cause me dissonance? What makes my body less than well?

> What behaviors should I implement before opting for a medical procedure or pharmaceuticals? What questions do I have for my doctor that I still have not asked?

> What behaviors have I concealed that my doctor needs to know to improve his/her service to me?

> Learn more about health risk assessments at: helpguide.org

Worksites: "Public and private employers and workplaces are included in this setting. Interventions may focus on the environments and policies that affect nutrition and physical activity in large and small workplaces and opportunities for employees to make healthful nutrition and physical activity choices."[11]

In every work industry, employers do their workforce a great justice by adding educational components to wellness efforts, including incentives for people to get moving and begin fueling their bodies healthfully.

WORKPLACE WELLNESS

While a positive workplace wellness culture can be developed through education, training, and incentive campaigns, we must also be aware of the social pressures that may enhance or diminish health. Professor of Business Law Robert A. Prentice lists the circumstances that often influence us to make poor nutrition and physical activity choices, both at work or at home:[12]

Obedience to Authority – to please authority we are likely to work longer hours and skimp on nutrition. Sometimes keeping our job depends on it.

Conformity Bias – cues from those around us push us to conform our judgment to the judgment of the group.

Incrementalism – refers to the "boiling frog" syndrome where a slow lowering of the bar of our behavior over time allows us to slip into unhealthy habits.

Groupthink – can lead us into poor decisions of all types.

Over Optimism – can lead to systematic errors in decision-making.

Over Confidence – can influence us to shortcut serious reflection about our behavior.

Self-Serving Bias – inclines us to gather information, process information, and remember information in such a way that it supports our preexisting views.

Framing – slick advertising can influence us to select a bag of chips labeled "95 percent fat free" rather than a bag labeled "5 percent fat" even though the chips are identical. Simply put, workplace persuasions appear in many forms and can be deviously powerful.

The Tangible, the Close, and the Near Term – most of us are more motivated by minor injuries to our own family than we are to genocide in foreign countries.

Loss Aversion – most people suffer losses twice as much as we enjoy gains; therefore we go to great lengths to avoid loss.

Learn how to build a workplace wellness culture at: bodyfactswellness.com

Prentice's list is long and somewhat disheartening, but as you have learned from reading this book, human beings are created with mirror neurons that automatically connect us with others who non-consciously influence us. The good news is that our bodies not only move us toward making wrong choices, they also move us toward making right ones.

This movement can be summarized in the following guide to experience all our senses—at work, at home, or in your community—through empathy:

See the despair that haunts others.

Hear the plea of our neighbors in need.

Smell the stench of poverty as well as the perfume of success.

Savor the taste of friendship.

Touch others by feeling love and compassion for them.

Our relational consciousness—our awareness that good to another is good to our self, and that harm to another is harm to our self—brings us full circle. Now we know that wellness in our Being Image is giving love to others. In fact, science has shown that philanthropy and kindness produces feel-good hormones and creates positive brain changes.

When we embrace life, we are brought into the fullness of our Being Image. When we develop three states of being: *informed, introspective,* and *intersubjective*—we can serve wellness in everything we think, say, and do. Then, we truly have Wellness in Mind.

As you get to know, celebrate, and share your Being Image, you appeal to the common character values of others, the actions of others, and the aspirations of others. You become an omnipotent influence that cuts through the distractions of life and upholds the dignity of all. The thick fabric of human connectivity—its symphony of courage, resilience, and endurance—allows for this highest-level communion.

As Charles Dickens has said, "No one is useless in this world who lightens the burdens of another." The best things in life are free: play, hugs, smiles, laughter, fellowship, acknowledgement, celebration, and gratitude.

Remember, when you're pointed in the right direction, baby steps are huge—start with a willing spirit and begin being.

You might be part of a whole Wellness Revolution!

APPENDIX: More of the Science Behind Wellness in Mind

Chapter 1

Mirror Neurons: Why We Imitate Others

Mirror neurons—first reported in the mid-1990s—are nerve cells that reside in specific anatomical areas of our brain. They fire when people watch mouth, hand, and foot movements and when they perform those actions (di Pellegrino et al. 1992; Gallese et al. 1996, 2002; Mukamel et al. 2010; Rizzolati et al. 1996). Thus, mirror neurons are thought to be bodily mediators of the coding for actions performed by the self and by another person (Gallese 2001, Rizzolatti & Craighero 2004).

What is going on is more than the preparation for and production of actions. What is going on is direct bodily understanding. Our direct bodily understanding, our automatic mirroring of each other, also includes recognizing, anticipating, predicting, and interpreting the actions of others. It is the way human beings directly understand another's intentions without thinking about them (Blakemore & Decety 2001).

Direct body understanding is called embodied simulation. Humans not only understand *what* others are doing but also *why* they are doing it. This is because when we see another do something, the mirror neurons in our brains activate "as if" we were performing the act even though we do not act. We experience in our brains and bodies what the other is doing. In one sense, when we've seen it, we've done it.

We also understand what others are feeling and sensing and *why* they are feeling and sensing. We call this capacity empathy. Neuroscientific studies suggest that empathy is underpinned by embodied simulation whereby we know another by activation of the same body-states underlying our own emotional and sensory experiences as what we observe in the other. When we've seen it, we've felt it.

Embodied simulation is possible because we are created with mirror neurons in our brains that enable our bodies to know another directly—body-to-body knowing. Human beings are interbodied in our knowing. We know each other bodily and directly before thinking, before introspection, before language. We know each other from within and directly when our own body-states associated with actions, emotions, and sensations are evoked by seeing another performing the actions or experiencing the emotions and sensations.

Of course, there is a difference between another and us. Even though mirror neurons fire both when an action or emotion is executed or perceived, the intensity of their firing is not the same. The intensity of the firing is greater when we actually do or feel something than when we merely see an action or emotion. Also, neuroanatomically different areas of our brain are activated. Studies show, for example, a difference in brain site activation between feeling disgust, imagining disgust, and observing another's facial expression of disgust (Jabbi et al. 2008).

The fact that we are created with mirror neurons in our brains means that we human beings are imitative beings. We cannot *not* imitate. We do it automatically, non-consciously. It is through imitation that we acquire language, culture, empathy, and our Being Image. Through our body-to-body knowing, we co-create one another.

It is vitally important, then, to be aware of who we imitate. It is equally important to know that the way we live will be imitated by others. We must strive to imitate and live wellness—to co-create wellness in others and in ourselves.

Attachment Patterns: How Relationships Organize Our Nervous System

During the past quarter-century of research, attachment theory has been the dominant approach to understanding the early social and emotional development of human beings. John Bowlby, a British medical doctor and psychoanalyst, defined and elaborated the concept of attachment. He proposed that human beings begin life with an inborn capacity that promotes attachment to their mother (Bowlby 1969). He viewed attachment seeking as instinctive social behavior with the biological function of maintaining proximity to a caregiver. Bowlby used his clinical observations of mother-child relationships to describe how these relationships become the means by which we bond to one another throughout life. Bowlby also introduced the idea of a "safe-base" (Bowlby 1973, 1988). When children feel safe in the presence of a sensitive and responsive caregiver, they experience a safe-base to play and explore their environment freely. This freedom is interrupted or impaired when children are not provided a safe-base.

Mary Ainsworth, Bowlby's associate, expanded Bowlby's view of attachment seeking by recognizing that children need not only proximity to caregivers but also emotional access in order to form attachment bonds. She further described that attachment seeking varied in intensity with perceived danger but always functioned to prevent separation from and to gain emotional access to a caregiver. For the scientific investigation of attachment seeking, Ainsworth invented a videotaped procedure (Ainsworth et al. 1978). This laboratory procedure, called the Strange Situation Test, made it possible to classify particular qualities of the attachment relationship between a child (twelve to twenty months of age—at the height of separation anxiety) and a caregiver. In the Strange Situation Test both child and caregiver play in a room supplied with toys until a friendly stranger (the experimenter) joins them. The caregiver then leaves the room, returns after three minutes, and resumes playing with her or his child and the experimenter. Then, both caregiver and experimenter leave. After another three minutes, the caregiver returns, which ends the experiment. Later, researchers view the taped situation and code the caregiver-child interactions, classifying the child according to one of three attachment patterns: secure attachment to his or her caregiver, insecure-avoidant attachment, or insecure-resistant attachment.

The secure attachment reflects a caregiver-child relationship that promotes well-being and serves as a source of resilience in stress. The caregiver's style of relating is one of being available to and effective with the child. The child's style of relating shows distress at the caregiver's departure, but comfort with their return. The reunion is a safe-base for the child freely to return to play. An insecure-avoidant attachment reflects a caregiver-child relationship that is impoverished. The caregiver's style of relating is one of being distant and rejecting. The child exhibits no overt distress when the caregiver leaves and on return, the child does not seek to be near the caregiver. An insecure-resistant attachment reflects a caregiver-child relationship where the caregiver is inconsistently available. The child exhibits distress even prior to the caregiver's leaving and is difficult to sooth and unable to play upon return. A safe-base has not been established with insecurely attached children.

A former student of Ainsworth, Mary Main, added a fourth category: disorganized/disoriented attachment (Main & Solomon 1986). A disorganized/disoriented attachment differs from the other three in that the other three attachments are organized. A disorganized/disoriented attachment is not organized and reflects a caregiver-child relationship in which the caregiver is a source of terror or alarm. The child is frightened by the caregiver's departure and shows contradictory behaviors upon their return. For example, the child may rise as if to go to the caregiver but instead falls prone to the floor. A safe-base is unavailable for these children.

Some children studied in the Strange Situation Test were followed up to the age of nineteen. Their original attachment pattern predicted subsequent behavior patterns, especially patterns of interpersonal relating with parents, teachers, and peers. It is as if their attachment pattern had become an internal working model by which they experienced others and life in general.

Interest then arose with regard to caregivers' attachment patterns. To study caregivers, Main, together with Eric Hesse, developed the Adult Attachment Interview. This semi-structured interview elicits a narrative of the adult's childhood memories of separations and losses, memories of illnesses, and memories of feelings such as feeling loved or unloved (Hesse

1999). Main and Hesse use a highly structured system to rate various aspects of the autobiographical narrative so that an adult can be classified reliably into attachment patterns. These attachment patterns both reflect how the adult bonded with his or her parents in the past and also predict how the adult will bond with his or her own children in the present or in the future, at least in contemporary Western culture (Belsky 2005).

Analysis of data from the Adult Attachment Interview revealed a group of people that have been called "earned" secure attachment. These are individuals with a history of insecure attachments, but whose adult interview narratives showed such flexibility in their reflective capacity that they were rated secure attachment. Their narratives suggest that they had formed a significant emotional relationship with someone, which allowed them to change from insecure attachment to secure attachment (Siegel 1999). Studies comparing "earned" secure and "continuous" secure, and insecure parents show no differences in the parent-child interactions of parents in the "earned" and "continuous" secure categories (Lichtenstein et al. 1998).

Building on the scientific discoveries in the attachment literature, we are coming to understand how our human nervous system is organized through relationship (Schore 2000b, Siegel 1999). Social attachment is a crucial motivator of behavior, which contributes to the development of attachment patterns that become internal working models of how we experience others and life in general (Mikulincer & Shaver 2010). Our neurophysiology depends on experiences in collaboration with others where we are learning *from* and *through* each other (Bråten 2007).

How we are I-Other: Intersubjectivity

Intersubjectivity—defined in the 1970s—is interpersonal communion. It is a *"sharing of experiential content (e.g. feelings, perceptions, thoughts, and linguistic meanings) among a plurality of subjects"* (Zlatev et al. 2008, 1). Intersubjectivity is made possible by our mirroring bodies. Human infants learn through direct resonance soon after birth (Bråten & Trevarthen 2007). When this direct resonance with another's expression of actions and emotions is a reciprocal subject-to-subject-sharing of psychobiological states rather than merely copying the other, the act has been named primary intersubjectivity.

Primary intersubjectivity is a dance-like proto-conversation that is observed as an infant's facial imitation of another's smile or tongue protrusion. An infant forty-two minutes old can express this innate tendency of all human beings to connect with another in dyadic engagement—in interactive action synchrony and affect attuning (Meltzoff 2011). "The 'function' of imitation might be its effect on the other and the interpersonal dialogue it promotes" (Reddy 2008, 65).

These mutual gaze communions are a central component in the formation of attachment bonds. Our mirror neuron mediated resonance allows infants to access their caregivers. The access is what attachment theorists view as essential for making contact and thriving. This motor and emotional attuning to others gives birth to our earliest sense of self—our bodily self (Gallese & Sinigaglia 2010). This body-to-body attuning shapes the self-experience of infant and other; it is a reciprocal interactive process.

Understood in this way, our earliest self is "an experienced self, understood only in-relation-to-the-other" (Reddy 2008, 143). Primary intersubjectivity operates at a pre-reflective (before thinking) motor and emotional intentionality. The motive for imitation seems to be firstly communication (beginning at birth) and secondly learning (beginning around the fifth month of life). As infants grow and develop, their capacity for intersubjectivity becomes increasingly complex.

Secondary intersubjectivity is where an object is the focus of joint attention and emotional referencing within a trusting relationship. It appears from about nine months of age. It is a triadic (infant, caregiver, and object) engagement of "cooperative awareness" (Trevarthen 2005, 70) of the world we share.

Tertiary intersubjectivity expresses collaborative engagement. It is attained in the second year of life when infants can engage in symbolic conversation, can share goals with others, and can share unspoken intentions. Sharing unspoken intentionality has been demonstrated in eighteen-month-old infants (Meltzoff 2011). Infants are shown adults successfully and unsuccessfully pulling an object apart. When the adult fails, the infants understand the adult's intention and complete the act of pulling the object apart. Infants are also shown an inanimate device successfully and unsuccessfully pulling an object apart. In the unsuccessful event, infants do not attribute intentions to the movements of the inanimate device and do not pull the object apart. With the attainment of tertiary intersubjectivity, thus, we can *share* the minds of others.

A fourth level of intersubjectivity—*understanding minds*—is achieved in year four of life (Allman et al. 2005). "This implicit and pre-theoretical, but at the same time contentful state enables us to directly understand what the other person is doing, why he or she is doing it, and how he or she feels about a specific situation" (Gallese 2011, 100). Once we can understand the minds of others, we have acquired a theory of mind (ToM). Having acquired a ToM, children can predict another's behavior based on intuiting attributes of the other's mental state.

In summary, mirror neurons mediate attuning that underpins imitation (an act of copying), intersubjectivity (an act of co-creating) and embodied simulation (the process supporting imitation and intersubjectivity). Intersubjectivity is the starting point for human development. "We are multiple [I-Other] from the start" (Haidt 2012, 109).

Chapter 2

Professional Credentials

Healthcare professionals recognize the important role physical activity plays in improving and maintaining good health. Unfortunately, the lack of professional credentials by some individuals working in fitness has slowed the acceptance of fitness professionals as legitimate members of the allied healthcare team by healthcare providers. As a result, the American Council on Exercise (ACE) and other top professional fitness organizations have earned third-party accreditation from the National Commission for Certifying Agencies (NCCA) for their fitness certification programs. For a complete list of NCCA-accredited fitness certifications organizations, visit www.credentialingexcellence.org.

Personal fitness trainers do not diagnose, prescribe, prescribe diets or recommend specific supplements, treat injury or disease, monitor progress for medically referred clients, rehabilitate, counsel, or work with patients.

In lieu of diagnosis, personal fitness trainers *do* receive exercise, health, or nutrition guidelines from a physician, physical therapist, registered dietitian, or other health professional, follow national consensus guidelines for exercise programming for medical disorders, screen for exercise limitations and identify potential risk factors, and refer clients to an appropriate allied health professional or medical practitioner.

In lieu of prescription, personal fitness trainers design exercise programs and refer clients to an appropriate allied health professional or medical practitioner for an exercise prescription.

In lieu of prescribing diets or recommending specific supplements, personal fitness trainers provide general information on healthy eating, according to the *MyPlate Food Guidance System* (United States Department of Agriculture: choosemyplate.gov) and refer clients to a dietician or nutritionist for a specific diet plan.

In lieu of treating injury or disease, personal fitness trainers refer clients to an appropriate allied healthcare professional or medical practitioner for treatment, use exercise to help improve overall health, and help clients follow physician or therapist advice.

In lieu of monitoring progress for medically referred clients, personal fitness trainers document progress, report to an appropriate allied health professional or medical practitioner, and follow physician, therapist, or dietitian recommendations.

In lieu of rehabilitation, personal fitness trainers design an exercise program once a client has been released from rehabilitation, coach, provide general information, and refer clients to a qualified counselor or therapist.

In lieu of working with *patients*, personal fitness trainers work with *clients*.

Chapter 3

Government Watchdogs

Government organizations that oversee health industries include the federal Centers for Disease Control and Prevention (CDC), the United States Department of Agriculture (USDA) and the Food and Drug Administration (FDA).

The role of the CDC is to protect the health security of our nation by responding to health threats, such as investigating local and nationwide outbreaks of foodborne illnesses. The CDC gathers data on foodborne outbreaks and monitors the effectiveness of prevention and control efforts in reducing foodborne illnesses. CDC also plays a key role in building state and local health department epidemiology, laboratory, and environmental health capacities to support foodborne disease surveillance and outbreak response.

The USDA has primary responsibility for the safety of meat, poultry, and certain egg products. The USDA's regulatory authority comes from the Federal Meat Inspection Act, the Poultry Products Inspection Act, the Egg Products Inspection Act, and the Humane Methods of Livestock Slaughter Act. The USDA inspects all meat, poultry, and egg products sold in interstate commerce and re-inspects imported meat, poultry, and egg products to make sure they meet U.S. safety standards. USDA continuously inspects slaughter facilities and examines each slaughtered meat and poultry carcass. USDA also visits every processing facility at least once during each operating day. In egg processing plants, the USDA inspects eggs before and after they are broken for further processing.

The FDA, as authorized by the federal Food, Drug and Cosmetic Act and the Public Health Service Act, regulates foods other than the meat and poultry products regulated by the USDA. FDA is also responsible for the safety of drugs, medical devices, vaccines, blood and biologics, animal and veterinary, cosmetics, tobacco products, and radiation emitting devices. Recently, the FDA Food Sa fety Modernization Act (FSMA) enables FDA to better protect public health by strengthening the food safety system. When this law goes into effect, the FDA will provide stricter oversight, ensure compliance with requirements and respond effectively when problems emerge.

To learn more about these important oversights visit fda.gov

The Acronym 3SP, A Note

As mentioned earlier, personal fitness trainers may not prescribe nutritional guidelines to clients. In accordance with this important boundary, the 3SP acronym derives from federal guidelines as published by the National Institute of Health, CDC and USDA.

We make no claim that the limitation of salt, sugar and saturated fat will result in weight-loss, reduce the chance of disease, increase health or increase performance. However, limitation and moderation decrease dependency on processed foods and increase the focus on live fare in the form of enjoyable natural foods. Fitness professionals must refer clients to a dietician or nutritionist for a specific diet plan (*American Council on Exercise Personal Trainer Manual* 2014).

Chapter 8

The Rotary Club: Andrew's Example of Engaged Citizenry In Action

My road to giving of myself rapidly widened when I accepted my father's invitation to join the world of Rotary in 1999. What is now called Rotary International began in Chicago in 1905 as a professional group that promoted fellowship. Its name derived from the practice of rotating meetings among members' offices; and helping others soon became its purpose.

The motto "Service Above Self" was expressed by its members in the voluntarily pooling of resources and contributions of talents to help serve communities in need. Today 1.2 million Rotarians belong to over 32,000 Rotary clubs in more than 200 countries.

In my experience, the spirit of Rotary exudes a commitment to the well-being of others. This is reflected in their goal to encourage and foster the ideal of service as a basis of worthy enterprise and, in particular, to encourage and foster:

First: The development of acquaintances as opportunities for service

Second: High ethical standards in business and professions, the recognition of the worthiness of all useful occupations, and the dignifying of each Rotarian's occupation as an opportunity to serve society

100

Third:	The application of the ideal of service in each Rotarian's personal and community life
Fourth:	The advancement of international understanding, goodwill, and peace through a world fellowship of business and professional persons united in the ideal of service

I particularly endorse the Four-Way Test of what Rotarians think, say, or do:

Is it the *truth*?
Is it *fair* to all concerned?
Will it build *goodwill* and *better friendships*?
Will it be *beneficial* to all concerned?

I solidified my personal stake in the health and wellness of Rotarians at the 2009 Rotary District 5520 conference in Ruidoso, New Mexico, where I attended the annual Sunday morning eulogy to Rotarians who passed away during the year. As a relatively young Rotarian, I had many older acquaintances and friends who suffered from health issues. When I opened the eulogy program to view names, I was shocked. Twenty-one Rotarians had died. This stark increase over previous years moved me toward my purpose of being. I decided to make an impact.

I volunteered to co-chair a district project that paired a blood drive called "Give a Pint" with a healthy weight drive. Indeed, the combination was renamed, "Give a Pint-Lose a Ton." The district gave twenty-nine pints of blood and lost a total of 687 pounds—not quite a ton, but enough to get Rotarians to think proactively about their health and well-being.

The next year, District 5520 shattered their goal to lose a ton with over 2,100 pounds lost! The challenge continued as a district program for two more years. During the 2013 conference, the District Wellness Committee offered a wellness education seminar and early morning Tai Chi with fellow Rotarian and committee co-chair, Mario DiJesu.

Rotary and its membership of business leaders may not be your niche in the realm of community service, so choose whichever philanthropic organization fits your personality best. Challenge your interrelatedness by providing for those more in need than you.

Wellness in Mind Activities

MY BEING IMAGE BLUEPRINT

1. Defining My Being Image

What are the values that are most important to you? Make a list.

2. Living My Being Image

What does living your Being Image look like? Define your vision of living in a state of wellness, in relation to the values you listed above. Describe what it looks like.

3. My Mission

Your mission becomes your purpose of being and the foundation of all your human interactions, such as, "I commit to upholding life values through the things I think, say and do." What is your mission?

HEALTHY-EATING SATISFACTION SURVEY

Hungry? Get specific about what you really crave by asking yourself the following questions:

What sounds the most appealing?

What looks the most appealing?

What taste am I craving (sweet, salty, or sour)?

What texture feels good (crunchy, crispy, or creamy)?

What smells appetizing?

When you're actually sitting down to your meal, try stopping after every three well-chewed bites and ask yourself:

How does my mind feel?

How does my chest cavity feel?

How does my stomach feel?

How do my extremities feel?

MY SMART GOALS

What are your movement and nourishment objectives? Specify your reasons for accomplishing these goals, their purpose, or benefits. Determine if your goal is to improve function, enrich health, increase fitness, or enhance performance. Now set three goals, making sure they are all clearly specific, measurable, achievable, relevant, and time-based.

GOAL #1:

GOAL #2:

GOAL# 3:

Now identify the strategies you need to use in order to reach these goals. What are the action items you plan to do?

Strategy 1: In order to achieve Goal 1, I must honor_____
_____every day.

Strategy 2: In order to achieve Goal 2, I must honor_____
_____every day.

Strategy 3: In order to achieve Goal 3, I must honor_____
_____every day.

MY SWOT ANALYSIS

STRENGTHS

Active engagement is the key to wellness. Your strengths will be found in your Life Line and Life Guards. Extract the character strengths from your Life Line that can help you achieve wellness.

What are my major life accomplishments?

What did I do great that helped me succeed?

What were the motivations and intentions for my victories?

Now list your Life Guards: the most important people in your life and the role models who have been paramount to your success.

Who are my major champions in life?

Who is teaching me something new?

For the rest of your SWOT analysis, use the six W questions (Who, What, When, Where, Why, and Which?) to take a look at:

WEAKNESSES

I. Who in my social circles is involved in unhealthy behaviors?
   Who is leading the charge? Who is aiding and abetting?
   Who can I influence using the life values of Family, Faith, Happiness and Health?
II. What unhealthy habits would I like to address?
   What unhealthy coping mechanisms are compounding my problems?
   What do people around me see as my weaknesses?
III. When do my unhealthy choices occur?
IV. Where do they occur?
V. Why do I fall back into a particular habit?
VI. Which of my perceived weaknesses can be reframed as strength?

OPPORTUNITIES

I. Who do I depend on daily? How can I honor my relationship with them?
II. What can I do to set the stage for servitude?

III. When is my energy level highest? When is it lowest?

IV. Where are the places I can learn and grow everyday?

V. Why not try something new today?

VI. Which dimensions of wellness can be enhanced right now?

THREATS

I. Who is troublesome or vexatious in my life? How can I help them?

II. What worries constitute idle time in my day?
What barriers do I face in my work?
What technologies threaten my wellness?

III. When do threats to my wellness occur?

IV. Where are unhealthy habits occurring most often?

V. Why have I allowed the burden of certain things or people to remain in my life?

VI. Which dimensions of my well-being do these threats attack?

MY BIG-PICTURE WORKSHEET

We'll be looking at each level of the Socio-Ecological Model one by one.

Myself as an Individual

Am I in harmony within my own self?
What blind spots, barriers, and burdens are impeding my success?
What are opportunities for growth with regard to knowledge, skills, attitudes, and beliefs?

I.   Who do I define myself as being?
II. What are my areas of knowledge, my attitudes, and my skills?
III. When and how often do thoughts about movement and play run through my mind?
IV. Where are the best opportunities for movement and play in my life?
V.   Why will maximizing my beingness benefit others: How will they benefit?
VI. Which of my wellness dimensions will be maximized as a result of being?

My Interpersonal Level

Am I in harmony within my family, friends, and social networks?
What blind spots, barriers, and burdens are impeding my success?
What are my opportunities?

I.   Who is a role model for me? How can I honor him/her?
II. What network of wellness champions do I have access to or can I create?
III. When are my social opportunities for growing my being?
IV. Where can I transform diminishing thoughts and behaviors into supportive love?
V.   Why, specifically, are my social networks important to me?
VI. Which dimension of wellness can best serve my interpersonal relationships?

My Organizational Level

Am I in harmony within my workplace and the social institutions I participate in?
What blind spots, barriers, and burdens are impeding my success?
What are my opportunities?

I. Who do I look up to? Who has the skills I want?
II. What technologies can help me move ahead?
III. When does my workplace best support my well-being?
IV. Where does my occupation best serve my wellness goals?
V. Why is it important to address workplace wellness at my work?
VI. Which best practices will help me model excellence?

My Community Level

Am I in harmony within relationships among the organizations I participate in?
What blind spots, barriers, and burdens are impeding my success?
What are my opportunities?

I. Who can I speak to about community wellness?
II. What needs in my company/industry are not being filled?
III. When can I reach into the community for advocates?
IV. Where is the most need?
V. Why are community wellness issues important for all?
VI. Which partnerships offer me the best chance to serve others?

My Public Policy Level

Am I in harmony within national, state, and local policies?
What public policy blind spots, barriers, and burdens are impeding success?
What are my opportunities?

I. Who is supportive of wellness in my neighborhood and voting precinct?
II. What are the pressing policy needs in my community?

III. When can we address policy needs?

IV. Where can I meet with policy stakeholders?

V. Why have certain wellness laws failed to serve the masses?

VI. Which lawmakers have a wellness focus? How can I access them?

Acknowledgements

M. Andrew Garrison

Wellness in Mind would have been impossible for me to write without Sally Severino. In the process of writing together, we listened to each other with a wish to understand and an openness to be changed by each other.

I want to acknowledge the woman I have always held in the most precious regard, the daughter who dreams big and loves to learn, and the son who reminds me daily that life is an honor: my wife Chamar, daughter Stefani, and son Blake. To my father, Dan Garrison, go my thanks for his guidance. To my second mother, Gaye Garrison, thanks for loving Dad so much and supporting my family in all our endeavors. Siblings Kathaleen and Phillip, I love you both—I am privileged to be close to you and your families.

My gratitude goes to my role models: Helen Garde, my teacher at Adobe Acres Elementary School, a lifelong friend whose compassion touched thousands of lives; Dora Gomez, my keyboarding teacher at Rio Grande High School, who comforted me when my mother died and modeled professionalism through her demeanor and consistent delivery; Coach Mike Sheppard, who gave me a second chance to play college football; and Dr. Leon Griffin, my university professor, who expanded my educational journey by recommending I pursue a masters degree in Sports Administration. His character and ethics sparked my continued pursuit of wellness knowledge.

Sally K. Severino

I met Andrew Garrison in 2012 at a monthly meeting of the SouthWest Writers Association. By chance, we sat at the same round table. I just happened to bring copies of my book *Sacred Desire: Growing in Compassionate Living.* Andrew thumbed through the book and said, "I'll buy this book on one condition." "What is the condition?" I asked. "That after I read your book, we get together and discuss it over a cup of coffee." "It's a deal," I agreed. It was over that cup of coffee that Andrew suggested we write a book together because he felt that my understanding of the psychobiosocial sciences as expressed in my book was consistent with his views about health and wellness. Excited by his proposal, we began our collaboration, which has grown into a cherished friendship.

We acknowledge with appreciation Cait Johnson for her suggestions, her editorial help, and her enthusiasm for this project. We thank our proofreaders, Joanne Caffrey and Annette De La Cruz, for their helpful input.

Additional thanks go to Lulu Publishing Services: to Logan Burton, Publishing/Marketing Consultant, who facilitated our Author Agreement process; to Adriane Pontecorvo, Check-In-Coordinator, who guided us through the submission and editorial process; to Carolyn Lockridge, Fulfillment Services Coordinator, who guided us through the rest of the publication process; and to the entire team who assisted these primary contacts.

Notes

1. WHAT IS BEING IMAGE, ANYWAY?

1   National Wellness Institute: https://nationalwellness.site-ym.com/?page=About Wellness.
2   National Wellness Institute: https://nationalwellness.site-ym.com/?page=Six_Dimensions.
3   Narvaez, D. (2014). *Neurobiology and the development of human morality: Evolution, culture, and wisdom.* New York: W.W. Norton & Company, p. 24.
4   Maslow, A. H. (1970). *Motivation and personality,* Second Edition. New York: Joanna Cotler Books.
5   Narvaez, 2014, Ibid., p. 24.
6   Rogoff, B. (2003). *The cultural nature of human development.* New York: Oxford University Press.
7   New Mexico Department of Health. (2006). "The New Mexico Plan to Promote Healthier Weigh 2006-2015," A Statewide Collaborative Coordinated by New Mexico Health and University of New Mexico Prevention Research Center, p. 3.
8   Morrison, N.K., & Severino, S. K. (2009). *Sacred desire: Growing in compassionate living.* West Conshohocken, PA: Templeton Foundation Press, p. 158.

2. MOVE IT!

1   Miller-Keane & O'Toole, M. T. (2005). *Encyclopedia and dictionary of medicine, nursing, and allied health,* Seventh Edition. St. Louis, MO: Saunders Company.
2   *American council on exercise health coach manual.* (2013). San Diego, CA: American Council on Exercise.
3   Csikszentmihalyi, M. (1996). *Creativity: The psychology of discovery and invention.* New York: HarperCollins Publishers.

3. NO MORE STARVING! FUEL YOURSELF WITH FOOD AND LOVE

[1]   Marketdata Enterprises, Inc. (February 2014). *The U.S. weight loss market: 2014 status report & forecast.* http://www.marketdataenterprises.com/

[2]   Institute of Medicine. (2005), *Strategies to reduce sodium intake in the United States.* Washington, DC: The National Academies Press.

[3]   Institute of Medicine. (2010). *Dietary reference intakes for water, potassium, sodium, chloride, and sulfate.* Washington, DC: The National Academies Press.

[4]   American Heart Association. http://www.heart.org/HEARTORG/Getting Healthy/NutritionCenter/HealthyDietGoals/Frequently-Asked-Questions-About-Sugar_UCM_306725_Article.jsp

[5]   Rolls, B. J. (1986). Sensory-specific satiety. *Nutrition Reviews*, 44, 93-101.

4. WELLNESS: IT'S ALL IN YOUR HEAD

[1]   Ansermet, F. & Magistretti, P. (2007). *Biology of freedom: Neural plasticity, experience, and the unconscious.* New York: Other Press.

[2]   Ibid., p. 195.

[3]   Schore, A. N. (2000a). Attachment and the regulation of the right brain. *Attachment and Human Development*, 2, 23-47.

[4]   Schore, A. N. (2000b). The self-organization of the right brain and the neurobiology of emotional development. In M. D. Lewis & I. Granic (Eds.). *Emotion, development, and self-organization* (pp. 155-185). New York: Cambridge University Press.

[5]   Morris, J. S., Öhman, A., & Dolan, R. J. (1999). A subcortical pathway to the right amygdala mediating unseen fear. *Proceedings of the National Academy of Science*, 96, 1680-1685.

[6]   Wikipedia: http://en.wikipedia.org/wiki/Cognitive_inertia.

[7]   Burns, D. (1980). *Feeling good: The new mood therapy.* New York: William Morrow.

[8]   Kitwood, T. (1990). *Concern for others: A new psychology of conscience and morality.* New York: Routledge.

[9]   Prochaska, J. O., DiClemente, C. C. & Norcross, J. C. (1992). In search of how people change. *American Psychologist*, 47, 1102-1114.

[10]   Velicer, W. F., Prochaska, J. O., Fava, J. L., et al. (1998). Smoking cessation and stress management: Applications of the Transtheoretical Model of behavior change. *Homeostasis*, 38, 216-233.

[11]   Prochaska et al. (1992), Ibid.

[12]   Velicer et al. (1998), Ibid.

6. REACH FOR RESILIENCE

1 Mate, G. (2010). *In the realm of hungry ghosts: Close encounters with addiction.* Berkeley, CA: North Atlantic Books, pp. 205-206.
2 Rahe, R. H., & Arthur, R. J. (1978). Life change and illness studies: Past history and future directions. *Journal Human Stress, 4,* 3-15.
3 Felitti, V. J., Anda, R. F., Nordenberg, D., et al. (1998). The relationship of adult health status to childhood abuse and household dysfunction. *American Journal of Preventive Medicine, 14,* 245-258.
4 Felitti, V. J., Anda, R. F. (2010). The relationship of adverse childhood experiences to adult medical disease, psychiatric disorders, and sexual behavior: Implications for healthcare. In R. A. Lanius, E. Vermetten, & C. Pain (Eds.), *The impact of early life trauma on health and disease: The hidden epidemic* (pp. 77-87). Cambridge, NY: Cambridge University Press.
5 Pfaff, D. W. (2007). *The neuroscience of fair play: Why we (usually) follow the golden rule.* New York: Dana Press, p. 56.
6 Doidge, N. (2015). *The brain's way of healing: Remarkable discoveries and recoveries from the frontiers of neuroplasticity.* New York: Viking.
7 Pfaff, 2007, Ibid., p. 36.
8 Perry, B. D. (2001). The neurodevelopmental impact of violence in childhood. In D. Schetky & E. Benedek (Eds.), *Textbook of child and adolescent forensic psychiatry* (pp. 221-238). Washington, DC: American Psychiatric Press.
9 Perry, B. D. & Szalavitz, M. (2006). *The boy who was raised as a dog: And other stories from a child psychiatrist's notebook.* New York: Basic Books, p. 249.
10 Morrison, N. K. & Severino, S. K. (2009). *Sacred desire: Growing in compassionate living.* West Conshohocken, PA: Templeton Foundation Press.

7. SERVING WELLNESS TO OTHERS

1 National Wellness Institute: https://nationalwellness.site-ym.com/?page=Six_Dimensions.
2 Alison, J. (2010). *Broken hearts & new creations: Intimations of a great reversal.* New York: Continuum, p. 62.
3 Thompson, G. & Jenkins, J. B. (2004). *Verbal judo: The gentle art of persuasion.* New Updated Edition. New York: William Morrow Paperbacks.

8. WELLNESS IN THE WORLD

1 Gergen, K. J. (2009). *Relational being: Beyond self and community.* New York: Oxford University Press.
2 Ibid., p. 397.

3   New Mexico Department of Health. (2006). "The New Mexico Plan to Promote Healthier Weight 2006-2015," A Statewide Collaborative Coordinated by New Mexico Health and University of New Mexico Prevention Research Center.

4   Ibid., p. 33.

5   Ibid., p. 36.

6   Ibid., p. 39.

7   Ibid., p. 42.

8   Chomsky, N. & Herman, E. (1988). *Manufacturing consent: The political economy of the mass media*. New York: Pantheon.

9   New Mexico Department of Health, 2006, Ibid., p. 44.

10 Deyle, G. D., MPT, Henderson, N. E. PhD, MPT, Matekel, R. L., MPT, et al. (2000). Effectiveness of manual physical therapy and exercise in osteoarthritis of the knee. *Annals of Internal Medicine, 132*(3), 173-181.

11 New Mexico Department of Health, 2006, Ibid., p. 46.

12 Prentice, R. A. (2007). Ethical decision making: More needed than good intentions. *Financial Analysts Journal, 63*(6), 17-30

References

Ainsworth, M. D. S., Blehar, M. C., Waters, E., et al. (1978). *Patterns of attachment: A psychological study of the strange situation.* Hillsdale, NJ: Lawrence Erlbaum.

Alison, J. (2010). *Broken hearts & new creations: Intimations of a great reversal.* New York: Continuum.

Allman, J. M., Watson, K. K., Tetreault, N. A., et al. (2005). Intuition and autism: A possible role for Von Economo neurons. *TRENDS in Cognitive Sciences, 9,* 367-373.

American council on exercise health coach manual. (2013). San Diego, CA: American Council on Exercise.

American council on exercise personal trainer manual. (2014). San Diego, CA: American Council on Exercise.

American Heart Association. http://www.heart.org/HEARTORG/ Getting_Healthy/NutritionCenter/HealthyDietGoals/Frequently-Asked-Questions-About-Sugar_UCM_306725_Article.jsp

Ansermet, F. & Magistretti, P. (2007). *Biology of freedom: Neural plasticity, experience, and the unconscious.* New York: Other Press.

Belsky, J. (2005). The developmental and evolutionary psychology of intergenerational transmission of attachment. In C. S. Carter, L. Ahnert, K. E. Grossman et al. (Eds.), *Attachment and bonding: A new synthesis* (pp. 169-198). Cambridge, MA: The MIT Press.

Blakemore, S-J, & Decety, J. (2001). From the perception of action to the understanding of intention. *Nature Reviews Neuroscience, 2,* 561-567.

Bowlby, J. (1969). *Attachment.* New York: Basic Books.

Bowlby, J. (1973). *Separation*. New York: Basic Books.

Bowlby, J. (1988). *A secure base: Parent-child attachment and healthy human development*. New York: Basic Books.

Bråten, S. (2007). *On being moved: From mirror neurons to empathy*. Philadelphia, PA: John Benjamins Publishing Company.

Bråten, S., & Trevarthen, C. (2007). Prologue: From infant intersubjectivity and participant movements to simulation and conversation in cultural common sense. In S. Bråten (Ed.), *On being moved: From mirror neurons to empathy* (pp. 21-34). Philadelphia, PA: John Benjamins Publishing Company.

Burns, D. (1980). *Feeling good: The new mood therapy*. New York: William Morrow.

Chomsky, N. & Herman, E. (1988). *Manufacturing consent: The political economy of the mass media*. New York: Pantheon.

Csikszentmihalyi, M. (1996). *Creativity: The psychology of discovery and invention*. New York: HarperCollins Publishers.

Deyle, G. D., MPT, Henderson, N. E. PhD, MPT, Matekel, R. L., MPT, et al. (2000). Effectiveness of manual physical therapy and exercise in osteoarthritis of the knee. *Annals of Internal Medicine, 132*(3), 173-181.

di Pellegrino, G., Fadiga, L., Fogassi, L., et al. (1992). Understanding motor events: A neurophysiological study. *Experimental Brain Research, 91*, 176-180.

Doidge, N. (2015). *The brain that changes itself: Remarkable discoveries and recoveries from the frontiers of neuroplasticity*. New York: Viking.

Felitti, V. J., Anda, R. F. (2010). The relationship of adverse childhood experiences to adult medical disease, psychiatric disorders, and sexual behavior: Implications for healthcare. In R. A. Lanius, E. Vermetten, & C. Pain (Eds.), *The impact of early life trauma on health and disease: The hidden epidemic* (pp. 77-87). Cambridge, NY: Cambridge University Press.

Felitti, V. J., Anda, R. F., Nordenberg, D., et al. (1998). The relationship of adult health status to childhood abuse and household dysfunction. *American Journal of Preventive Medicine, 14*, 245-258.

Gallese, V. (2001). The "shared manifold" hypothesis: From mirror neurons to empathy. *Journal of Consciousness Studies, 8*, 33-50.

Gallese, V. (2011). The two sides of mimesis: Mimetic theory, embodied simulation, and social identification. In S. R. Garrels (Ed.), *Mimesis and science: Empirical research on imitation and the mimetic theory of culture and religion* (pp. 87-108). East Lansing, MI: Michigan State University Press.

Gallese, V., Fadiga, L, Fogassi, L., et al. (1996). Action recognition in the premotor cortex. *Brain, 119,* 593-609.

Gallese, V., Fadiga, L., Fogassi, L., et al. (2002). Action representation and the inferior parietal lobule. In W. Prinz & B. Hommel (Eds.), *Attention and performance XIX: Common mechanisms in perception and action* (pp. 334-355). New York: Oxford University Press.

Gallese, V., & Sinigaglia, C. (2010). The bodily self as power for action. *Neuropsychologia, 48,* 746-755.

Gergen, K. J. (2009). *Relational being: Beyond self and community.* New York: Oxford University Press.

Haidt, J. (2012). *The righteous mind: Why good people are divided by politics and religion.* New York: Pantheon Books.

Hesse, E. (1999). The adult attachment interview: Historical and current perspectives. In J. Cassidy & P. Shaver (Eds.), *Handbook of attachment: Theory, research, and clinical applications* (pp. 395-433). New York: Guilford.

Institute of Medicine. (2005), *Strategies to reduce sodium intake in the United States.* Washington, DC: The National Academies Press.

Institute of Medicine. (2010). *Dietary reference intakes for water, potassium, sodium, chloride, and sulfate.* Washington, DC: The National Academies Press.

Jabbi, M., Bastiaansen, J., & Keysers, C. (2008). A common anterior insula representation of disgust observation, experience and imagination shows divergent functional connectivity pathways. *PLoS ONE:* e2939. doi:10.1371/journal.pone.0002939.

Kitwood, T. (1990). *Concern for others: A new psychology of conscience and morality.* New York: Routledge.

Lichtenstein P. J., Belsky, J. & Crnic, K. (1998). Earned security, daily stress, and parenting: A comparison of five alternative models. *Development and Psychopathology, 10*: 21-38.

Longley, R. (August 22, 2010). *The US food satiety system: A case of shared government responsibilities.* http://usgovinfo.about.com/od/consumerawareness/a/The-Us-Food-Safety-System:htm

Main, M. & Solomon, J. (1986). Discovery of an insesure-disorganized/disoriented attachment pattern. In T. B. Brazelton & M. Yogman (Eds.), *Affective development in infancy,* (pp. 95-124). Norwood, NJ: Ablex.

Marketdata Enterprises, Inc. (May 1, 2011). *U.S. weight loss & diet control market,* 11th Edition. http://www.marketdataenterprises.com/

Maslow, A. H. (1970). *Motivation and personality,* Second Edition. New York: Joanna Cotler Books.

Mate, G. (2010). *In the realm of hungry ghosts: Close encounters with addiction.* Berkeley, CA: North Atlantic Books.

Meltzoff, A. N. (2011). Out of the mouths of babes: Imitation, gaze, and intentions in infant research—the "like me" framework. In S. R. Garrels (Ed.). *Mimesis and science: Empirical research on imitation and the mimetic theory of culture and religion* (pp. 55-74). East Lansing, MI: Michigan State University Press.

Mikulincer, M. & Shaver, P. R. (2010). *Attachment in Adulthood: Structure, Dynamics, and Change.* New York: The Guilford Press.

Miller-Keane & O'Toole, M. T. (2005). *Encyclopedia and dictionary of medicine, nursing, and allied health,* Seventh Edition. St. Louis, MO: Saunders Company.

Morris, J. S., Öhman, A., & Dolan, R. J. (1999). A subcortical pathway to the right amygdala mediating unseen fear. *Proceedings of the National Academy of Science, 96,* 1680-1685.

Morrison, N.K., & Severino, S. K. (2009). *Sacred desire: Growing in compassionate living.* West Conshohocken, PA: Templeton Foundation Press.

Mukamel, R., Ekstrom, A. D., Kaplan J., et al. (2010). Single-neuron responses in humans during execution and observance of actions. *Current Biology, 20,* 750-756.

Narvaez, D. (2014). *Neurobiology and the development of human morality: Evolution, culture, and wisdom.* New York: W.W. Norton & Company.

National Wellness Institute: https://nationalwellness.site-ym. com/?page=About Wellness.

National Wellness Institute: https://nationalwellness.site-ym. com/?page=Six_Dimensions.

New Mexico Department of Health. (2006). "The New Mexico Plan to Promote Healthier Weight 2006-2015," A Statewide Collaborative Coordinated by New Mexico Health and University of New Mexico Prevention Research Center.

Perry, B. D. (2001). The neurodevelopmental impact of violence in childhood. In D. Schetky & E. Benedek (Eds.), *Textbook of child and adolescent forensic psychiatry* (pp. 221-238). Washington, DC: American Psychiatric Press.

Perry, B. D. & Szalavitz, M. (2006). *The boy who was raised as a dog: And other stories from a child psychiatrist's notebook*. New York: Basic Books.

Pfaff, D. W. (2007). *The neuroscience of fair play: Why we (usually) follow the golden rule*. New York: Dana Press.

Prentice, R. A. (2007). Ethical decision making: More needed than good intentions. *Financial Analysts Journal, 63*(6), 17-30.

Prochaska, J. O., DiClemente, C. C. & Norcross, J. C. (1992). In search of how people change. *American Psychologist, 47*, 1102-1114.

Rahe, R. H., & Arthur, R. J. (1978). Life change and illness studies: Past history and future directions. *Journal Human Stress, 4*, 3-15.

Reddy, V. (2008). *How infants know minds*. Cambridge, MA: Harvard University Press.

Rizzolatti, G., & Craighero, L. (2004). The mirror-neuron system. *Annual Review Neuroscience, 27*, 169-192.

Rizzolati, G., Fadiga, L., Gallese, V., et al. (1996). Premotor cortex and the recognition of motor actions. *Cognitive Brain Research, 3*, 131-141.

Rogoff, B. (2003). *The cultural nature of human development*. New York: Oxford University Press.

Rolls, B. J. (1986). Sensory-specific satiety. *Nutrition Reviews, 44*, 93-101.

Schore, A. N. (2000a). Attachment and the regulation of the right brain. *Attachment and Human Development, 2*, 23-47.

Schore, A. N. (2000b). The self-organization of the right brain and the neurobiology of emotional development. In M. D. Lewis & I.

Granic (Eds.). *Emotion, development, and self-organization* (pp. 155-185). New York: Cambridge University Press.

Siegel, D. J. (1999). *The developing mind: Toward a neurobiology of interpersonal experience*. New York: Guilford.

Thompson, G. & Jenkins, J. B. (2004). *Verbal judo: The gentle art of persuasion*, New Updated Edition. New York: William Morrow Paperbacks.

Trevarthen, C. (2005). "Stepping away from the mirror: Pride and shame in adventures of companionship"—reflections on the nature and emotional needs of infant intersubjectivity. In C. S. Carter, L. Ahnert, K. E. Grossman, et al. (Eds.), *Attachment and bonding: A new synthesis* (pp. 55-84). Cambridge, MA: The MIT Press.

Velicer, W. F., Prochaska, J. O., Fava, J. L., et al. (1998). Smoking cessation and stress management: Applications of the Transtheoretical Model of behavior change. *Homeostasis*, *38*, 216-233.

Wikipedia: http://en.wikipedia.org/wiki/Cognitive_inertia.

Zlatev, J., Racine, T. P., Sinha, C., et al. (2008). Intersubjectivity: What makes us human? In J. Zlatev, T. P. Racine, C. Sinha, et al. (Eds.), *The shared mind: Perspectives in intersubjectivity* (pp. 1-14). Philadelphia, PA: John Benjamins Publishing Company.